P9-BIV-764

WHOLESOME DIET

*This volume is one of a series designed to familiarize readers
with the latest advances in medical science and to guide them in
maintaining their own health and fitness.*

WHOLESOME DIET

BY THE EDITORS OF TIME-LIFE BOOKS

LIBRARY OF HEALTH / TIME-LIFE BOOKS / ALEXANDRIA, VIRGINIA

THE CONSULTANT:

Dr. Myron Winick is Director of the Institute of Human Nutrition and the Center for Nutrition, Genetics and Human Development at Columbia University's College of Physicians and Surgeons in New York City, where he also serves as professor of nutrition and pediatrics. Dr. Winick is the author of *Malnutrition and Brain Development* and the editor of nine volumes in the series *Current Concepts in Nutrition*.

For information about any Time-Life book, please write:
Reader Information, Time-Life Books,
541 North Fairbanks Court, Chicago, Illinois 60611.

First printing.
Published simultaneously in Canada.
School and library distribution by Silver Burdett Company, Morristown, New Jersey.

TIME-LIFE is a trademark of Time Incorporated U.S.A.

Library of Congress Cataloguing in Publication Data
The Editors of Time-Life Books
    Wholesome Diet
    (Library of Health)
    Bibliography: p.
    Includes index.
    1. Nutrition.   2. Diet.
    I. Time-Life Books. II. Title. III. Series.
RA784.W613   613.2   81-8987
ISBN 0-8094-3768-6   AACR2
ISBN 0-8094-3767-8 (lib. bdg.)
ISBN 0-8094-3766-X (retail ed.)

59,983

Time-Life Books Inc. is a wholly owned subsidiary of

TIME INCORPORATED

FOUNDER: Henry R. Luce 1898-1967

Editor-in-Chief: Henry Anatole Grunwald
President: J. Richard Munro
Chairman of the Board: Ralph P. Davidson
Executive Vice President: Clifford J. Grum
Chairman, Executive Committee: James R. Shepley
Editorial Director: Ralph Graves
Group Vice President, Books: Joan D. Manley
Vice Chairman: Arthur Temple

TIME-LIFE BOOKS INC.

MANAGING EDITOR: Jerry Korn
Executive Editor: David Maness
Assistant Managing Editors: Dale M. Brown (planning), George Constable, Martin Mann, John Paul Porter, Gerry Schremp (acting)
Art Director: Tom Suzuki
Chief of Research: David L. Harrison
Director of Photography: Robert G. Mason
Assistant Art Director: Arnold C. Holeywell
Assistant Chief of Research: Carolyn L. Sackett
Assistant Director of Photography: Dolores A. Littles

CHAIRMAN: John D. McSweeney
President: Carl G. Jaeger
Executive Vice Presidents: John Steven Maxwell, David J. Walsh
Vice Presidents: George Artandi (comptroller); Stephen L. Bair (legal counsel); Peter G. Barnes; Nicholas Benton (public relations); John L. Canova; Beatrice T. Dobie (personnel); Carol Flaumenhaft (consumer affairs); James L. Mercer (Europe/South Pacific); Herbert Sorkin (production); Paul R. Stewart (marketing)

LIBRARY OF HEALTH

Editorial Staff for *Wholesome Diet*
Editor: William Frankel
Assistant Editor: Phyllis K. Wise
Designer: Albert Sherman
Picture Editor: Jane Speicher Jordan
Text Editors: Laura Longley Babb, Brian McGinn, C. Tyler Mathisen, David Thiemann
Staff Writer: Peter Kaufman
Researchers: Judy French, Judith Shanks (principals), Jean Crawford, Barbara Hicks, Norma Kennedy, Sara Mark, Fran Moshos, Rita Mullin, Trudy Pearson, Jules Taylor
Assistant Designer: Cynthia T. Richardson
Editorial Assistant: Nana Heinbaugh Juarbe
Special Contributors: Writers: Ann Aikman, Susan Perry, Arthur Fisher, Phyllis Lehmann, Wendy Murphy, Lydia Preston, Jane Stein; Researchers: Sharon Block, Mindy Daniels, Barbara Lerner, David F. Long

EDITORIAL PRODUCTION
Production Editor: Feliciano Madrid
Operations Manager: Gennaro C. Esposito, Gordon E. Buck (assistant)
Quality Control: Robert L. Young (director), James J. Cox (assistant), Daniel J. McSweeney, Michael G. Wight (associates)
Art Coordinator: Anne B. Landry
Copy Staff: Susan B. Galloway (chief), Margery duMond, Stephen G. Hyslop, Diane Ullius Jarrett, Celia Beattie
Picture Department: Rebecca C. Christoffersen
Traffic: Kimberly K. Lewis

Correspondents: Elisabeth Kraemer, Helga Kohl (Bonn); Margot Hapgood, Dorothy Bacon, Lesley Coleman (London); Susan Jonas, Lucy Voulgaris (New York); Maria Aloisi, Josephine du Brusle (Paris); Ann Natanson (Rome). Valuable assistance was also given by: Janny Hovinga, Wibo Van De Linde (Amsterdam); Dick Rose (Arizona); Nina Lindley (Buenos Aires); Katrina Van Duyn (Copenhagen); Lance Keyworth, Risto Maenpaa (Helsinki); Peter Hawthorne (Johannesburg); Judy Aspinall, Jeremy Lawrence, Karin Pearce, Pippa Pridham (London); Cheryl Crooks (Los Angeles); Carolyn Chubet, Miriam Hsia, Christina Lieberman (New York); Bent Onsager (Oslo); John Scott (Ottawa); Mimi Murphy, Ann Wise (Rome); Janet Zich (San Francisco); Mary Johnson (Stockholm); Edwin Reingold, Eiko Fukuda, Frank Iwama, Michiko Koga (Tokyo); Traudl Lessing (Vienna).

CONTENTS

CHAPTER 1

The staffs of life

Meeting the basic needs
Penalties of abundance
The great Protein Shift
Perils in production-line food
Meals of mystical power
A banquet of elixirs

For more than 2,000 years, authorities have been giving advice on what, how and when to eat. For at least as long, many people have ignored the advice and trusted their own instincts—and taste buds—to guide them in choosing the right foods. "If the physician and the cook," wrote the Greek philosopher Plato in the Fourth Century B.C., "had to enter into a competition as to which of them best understands the goodness or badness of food, the physician would be starved to death." Twenty centuries later, the French philosopher Montesquieu registered his own complaint about nutritional advice. "The kind of health," he wrote in the 17th Century, "that can be preserved only by a careful and constant regulation of diet is but a tedious disease."

Controversies over diet rage today more fiercely than ever. People everywhere are bombarded with often-conflicting advice from government agencies, health associations, insurance companies and teachers. Rumors—occasionally substantiated—that modern processing and preserving techniques are poisoning food frighten many. For some, eating has turned into a game of nutritional roulette. Others, convinced that modern farming methods rob foods of vital ingredients, resort to enormous doses of vitamin and mineral supplements to compensate for supposedly missing nutrients. And health-food enthusiasts, persuaded that their ancestors were healthier than contemporary humans, adopt the dietary and farming practices of earlier societies in the hope of avoiding the diseases they associate with modern diets.

The confusion is understandable in a time of rapid change.

Very few people in the industrialized world eat the same kinds of foods their grandparents—perhaps even their parents—ate. The reassurance of centuries of experience with traditional foods is lost. And there is much evidence that departures from traditional foodstuffs and methods have brought harm as well as benefits.

Industrial revolutions have shifted entire populations from country to city and changed the nature of work from back-breaking farm labor to sedentary factory or office occupations. Canning and refrigeration have made it possible to preserve for year-round use foods that were formerly available for only a month or two each year. Transportation networks have made it possible to move food safely and cheaply from coast to coast or from one country to another, increasing shoppers' choices to the more than 12,000 products that are available in the modern supermarket. Today, science and technology continue to change the shape, taste, texture, color and even the content of food—sometimes to advantage, sometimes not.

A large part of the confusion also stems from the fact that the science of nutrition itself is still in its infancy. Discoveries and advances in many fields of knowledge have led to radical swings in nutritional theories and advice. Like any evolving science that makes an attempt to deal with the bewildering variability of the human species, the study of nutrition has suffered from its share of premature conclusions and outright errors.

Even elaborate and carefully planned and executed re-

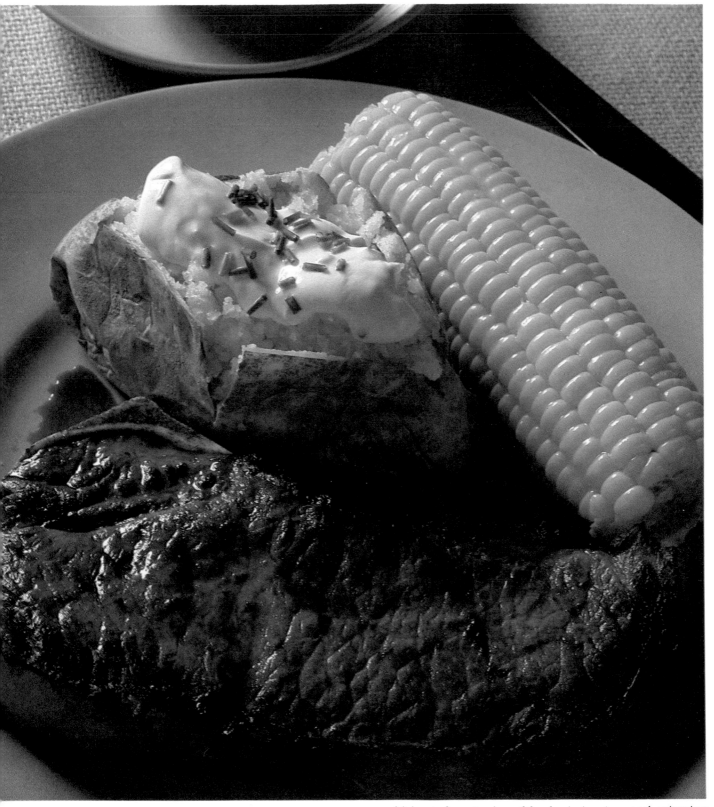

A juicy steak, centerpiece of the classic American meal, epitomizes the surplus of fat in most Western diets. This 12-ounce cut of beef alone contains more than four times the average daily need for fat. Add the fat contributed by sour cream on the potato, and butter on the corn, and this hearty plateful helps build a diet that can lead to obesity and heart disease.

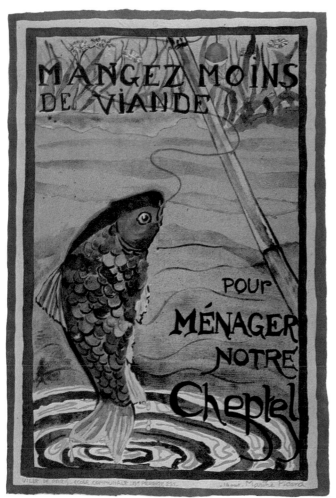

A fisherman's prize catch highlights a World War I poster exhorting the people of France to ''eat less meat to conserve our livestock.'' The war-caused shift from meat to fish offered another benefit then unrecognized—fish contains less of the fats implicated in circulatory ailments and cancer.

search can lead to dubious advice. A study that followed almost 7,000 people in Alameda County, California, over a period of five years found a higher death rate among those who did not eat breakfast regularly. That finding was used to support one of the traditional rules for a healthful diet: Eat a good breakfast.

This edict aroused the skepticism of Dr. Lewis Thomas, a renowned biologist and commentator, and the Chancellor of the Memorial Sloan-Kettering Cancer Center in New York City. ''Among the people who answered that they don't eat breakfast,'' he wrote, ''there were surely some who were already ill when the questionnaire arrived. They didn't eat breakfast because they couldn't stand the sight of food. They had lost their appetites, were losing weight, didn't feel up to moving around much, and had trouble sleeping. Some of these people probably had an undetected cancer; others may have had hypertension or early kidney failure or some other organic disease which the questionnaire had no way of picking up.'' Concluded Dr. Thomas: ''It is hard to imagine any good reason for dying within five years from not eating a good breakfast, or any sort of breakfast.''

Amid all the debates there are many areas of agreement. From the abundance of foods made available to much of the world by modern farming and processing, the most wholesome can be selected and the suspect minority avoided. The risks attending the use of vitamin and mineral supplements, some additives and preservatives, and certain reducing diets are better known now; they can be weighed against real benefits so that individual choices are possible. The burgeoning evidence of the dangers from obesity and from overreliance on some types of food suggests modifications in diet that will protect and prolong life. Deeper understanding of the physiological effects of foods has identified some that prevent disease and others that cause it.

Meeting the basic needs

Accurate knowledge about diet has been a long time coming. Not until 1827 did the English chemist William Prout venture the notion that all living things needed at least three nutrients: ''the saccharine, the oily and albuminous.'' By 1846 the

German chemist Baron Justus von Liebig had proved that three classes of compounds were indeed utilized by the human body, and they corresponded roughly with Prout's list: carbohydrates, mainly from plants; fats from plants and animals; and proteins, present in some plants but obtained mainly by the consumption of animal foods—meat, poultry, fish, eggs, milk and cheese. More recent research has proved that other substances also are needed, in smaller quantities: the complex compounds called vitamins and the elemental minerals such as iron and calcium.

These essential ingredients can be supplied by an amazing variety of foods. Around the world, different peoples eat different foods, and no particular diet has proved ideal. So long as there is enough to eat, almost everyone everywhere, regardless of the technology of the culture or the particular foods it provides, gets enough of the necessary nutrients to maintain adequate health. Many people do amazingly well with resources that may seem meager.

In Mexico the dietary staple is corn, a grain that yields more food value per acre of cropland than any other. But corn lacks some substances that humans need. The Mexicans make up for the missing ingredients by eating with their corn black beans, pork, chicken, cheese, fruits, vegetables and chili peppers. Trial and error over the millennia has also shown them how to increase the nutritive value of cornmeal by soaking it in a limestone solution before baking it into tortillas. The process results in a 20-fold increase in the corn's content of the important nutrient calcium, obtained elsewhere from dairy products (in Mexico, dairying hardly existed as an industry until recent years).

In China, cooks discovered ingenious ways to harness the great nutritive value locked in the soybean, which when raw is not only indigestible but poisonous. The beans can be rendered harmless and digestible by prolonged cooking, but the fuel needed is scarce in China. The Chinese learned several other methods for converting soybeans into safe, nutritious food: germinating the soybeans into edible bean sprouts, fermenting them into soy sauce, or steaming them into bean curd—a process that requires relatively small amounts of fuel.

In the frozen wastes of the Canadian Arctic, early Eskimos managed to obtain adequate nutrition by scouring the wilderness for a wide variety of animal and plant foods. Explorers reported that the Eskimos subsisted on an exclusive diet of caribou, seal and animal fats in such forms as whale blubber. The reports puzzled scientists, for a meat diet lacks essential ingredients found only in plant foods. Later investigations revealed that the Eskimos supplemented their meat staple by gathering berries, roots and willow buds. In addition, they ate as a delicacy the stomach contents of the plant-eating animals they hunted.

The very complexity of diets such as the Eskimos' made them healthful; eating a wide variety of foods lessens the chance that any essential nutrients will be lacking. Such variety was not always available to hunter-gatherers, impoverished farmers or the city poor. For all but the wealthy few in Europe and America, the daily fare was monotonous meals of bread, potatoes, butter and cheese, supplemented by an occasional bit of salted beef or smoked pork. As a result, deficiency diseases were common. Poor rural communities in southern Europe and the southeastern United States were long plagued by debilitating pellagra, and in cities all over the world children exhibited the stunted bones and bowed legs of rickets.

Penalties of abundance

Today, deficiency diseases are practically unknown in the industrialized world. Only scattered pockets of hunger persist, as a generally high standard of living permits almost everyone to get enough to eat and to select from a vast array of foods. The old concerns are gone—but they have been replaced by new ones, all the more frustrating because they are peculiar to the 20th Century.

In the more affluent industrialized countries, the achievement of affluence itself has skewed diets. The sheer abundance of food in the United States, Canada, Japan and Western Europe has proved a mixed blessing. Many people eat more than their bodies need, with the result that overweight afflicts one in every three Americans, is the most common nutritional defect in the industrialized countries, and helps account for the great plagues of the modern world: high blood pressure, heart disease, kidney disease, circulatory disease, diabetes and cancer. "Death on the expense account," commented the microbiologist René Dubos, "is a characteristic feature of the affluent society."

Overnutrition is new only in its prevalence. "Human beings," wrote Dubos, "always have been prone to overcompensate for fear of food shortages by engaging in nutritional excesses whenever they could afford it." Perhaps the best example of such dietary indulgence is the eating practices of the ancient Romans.

Like many modern-day executives, Roman patricians ate sparingly during the day. A typical breakfast consisted only of a drink of water or wine, and lunch was usually just a snack. In the evenings, however, all self-control was abandoned. Dinner was a sumptuous, multicourse formal banquet and included exotic foods and spices imported from every corner of the Empire. There were sausages from Greece, oysters from Britain, hams from Gaul, pickles from Spain, pomegranates from Libya, and wines from the Jura region of Switzerland.

Although there is little reliable medical evidence of the effects of this rich diet, ancient literature provides some clues. "Overfeeding," warned an old Roman proverb, "destroys more than hunger." And the poet Lucretius put the matter even more bluntly. Speaking of earlier times, he wrote: "In those days it was lack of food that drove fainting bodies to death; now contrariwise it is the abundance that overwhelms them."

In Rome, at least, the effects of this abundance were confined to the upper classes; the average person got by on a bland diet of coarse bread and gruel. Nowadays, however, almost everyone shares both the fruits and the problems of abundance. And the very technology that has made food available in such quantities the year round has also introduced another cause of the diseases of abundance. Obesity fundamentally arises from eating too much and exercising too little. During the past century, machines have assumed most of the tasks that were previously performed by human muscles. Automobiles have largely eliminated walking, and

elevators have made stair-climbing practically unnecessary. Laborsaving devices have taken over many of the manual tasks of the workplace, creating more and more sedentary occupations for human beings. Nowadays even a ditchdigger is a skilled technician who digs ditches while sitting down, expending no more effort than is required to manipulate the controls of his machine.

This decrease in exercise, however, has not been matched by a corresponding decrease in appetites. Since 1910, when most Americans were still engaged in manual labor, the total intake of food per capita has fallen by only 3 per cent. But life has become so sedentary in the interim that 97 per cent of the 1910 diet is far too much food. Many modern-day executives, chairbound from nine till five, still consume dinners designed for a turn-of-the-century farmer who worked in the fields from dawn to dusk. "What was adequate nutrition yesterday," wrote Dubos, "is probably overnutrition—and also malnutrition—today."

The introduction of central heating and air-conditioning systems, which have made life more healthful and pleasant in many areas, has also changed dietary needs in a more subtle manner. Previously, people who lived in cold and damp climates had a practical reason to put on an extra layer of fat: It served to insulate their bodies from the weather. Nowadays, central heating systems protect from the extremes of climate and make added fat a potentially dangerous holdover from the past.

The great Protein Shift

Affluence alters not only the quantity of food consumed but also the type. People everywhere switch from cereal foods such as bread, pasta and rice to animal foods whenever they can. This phenomenon, which economists have dubbed the "Protein Shift," occurs when improvements in the general standard of living make meat affordable to a large part of the population. Eleven of the more developed countries account for a staggering 40 per cent of the world's total meat consumption. In those countries, the cereal grains are fed to livestock. The animals convert cereal carbohydrates into proteins, and people eat the proteins in their meat.

The Protein Shift brings both benefits and dangers. Animal protein derived from meat is a rich source of needed nutrients. But increased meat consumption has been closely linked to heart disease. Many meats, in addition to serving as excellent protein sources, also contain appreciable amounts of animal fats, which apparently harm blood vessels. The effect is measurable everywhere; it is especially obvious in Japan, where for many years the average diet contained very little meat and between 66 and 75 per cent less fat than was eaten in most other countries. After World War II, Japan's industrial affluence permitted its people to increase their consumption of meat—and the nation's death rate from heart disease leaped upward by approximately 20 per cent between 1940 and 1967.

Although overindulgence in meat may bring some hazard, no one should try to follow the advice of Wilbur Olin Atwater, a 19th Century chemist who advised housewives not to bother buying meat—or fresh fruit and vegetables. Atwater was a brilliant researcher who made important contributions to nutritional science, but he somehow reached the conclusion that the cheaper sources of food energy, such as breads and cereals, were just as good as the more expensive meats and fresh produce. They are not.

Perils in production-line food

At the same time the Protein Shift was reducing the amount of carbohydrates that were eaten, the kinds eaten were also undergoing a change. The 20th Century has brought a decrease in the consumption of so-called complex carbohydrate foods such as fresh fruits, vegetables and whole-grain breads. There has been a corresponding increase in the consumption of simple carbohydrates, which include sugar and honey. The latter group does provide food energy measured in calories, but the calories are nutritionally empty—they contain none of the vitamins, minerals and fiber that are found in the complex carbohydrates.

One of the more notable victims of this switch has been the potato, a highly nutritious vegetable that is rich in many vitamins as well as the mineral iron. Potatoes also retain most of their nutrients even after months in storage so that they

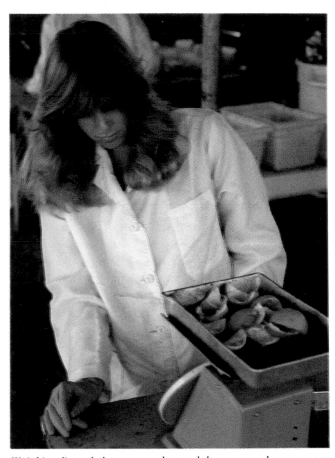

Weighing discarded orange peels on a laboratory scale, a University of Arizona student takes part in a project monitoring the food waste of some 7,000 Tucson households by analyzing their garbage. The study compared the weight of the waste with its average original weight and concluded that about 15 per cent of the food Tucson's half million residents threw out each day— a total of some 10,000 tons a year—was still edible.

are readily available year-round—and they are inexpensive.

Despite these highly desirable properties, potatoes have acquired a reputation as a fattening food, probably as a result of the fashionable low-carbohydrate reducing diets. The reputation is unjustified. Ounce for ounce, a potato is about as fattening as an apple or a pear. Nevertheless, many weight-conscious people will push aside a potato while they are digging into a steak, which—even when the visible fat has been trimmed off—is four to five times more fattening than the potato.

Such a transformation of eating practices would have been impossible without the revolution in food processing that began in the 19th Century and accelerated in the 20th. Canned, frozen and refined products now account for 55 per cent of the average American diet. These foods make possible unprecedented variety, but some of the nutrients are lost during processing, and chemical additives and preservatives, as well as nonnutritious carbohydrates such as sugar, are added. A preference for processed foods, like the taste for protein and sweets, seems to be almost universal whenever affluence permits.

From the time of the Egyptians and the Romans, for example, white bread has been a status food closely associated with wealth and well-being, while the coarser and darker breads were reserved for the poorer classes. Most people think that white bread tastes better. Similarly, white rice has been the status food in the Orient, while brown rice was eaten only by those who could not afford the polished, lighter-colored variety.

The poorer classes were getting the better nutrition. Whole-grain flour contains more vitamins and minerals than the highly refined type, and brown rice is rich in a vitamin that prevents the disease beriberi.

Roman millers went to great lengths to whiten flour for their aristocratic patrons. After grinding the wheat between stones, they sieved, or bolted, the coarse mixture through cloths to remove the dark-colored outer husk called the bran. Then they added a special chalky substance called *creta* to whiten the residue. "In order of merit," wrote the Roman hygienist Diphilus of Siphnos, in the Fourth Century B.C.,

"the bread made from refined flour comes first, after that bread of ordinary wheat, and then the unbolted, made from flour that has not been sifted."

As recently as the 18th Century, millers and bakers were still adding chalk, bone ash and alum to flour. Still, wheat flour retained a characteristic yellowish hue, even after the bran was removed. The color was caused by the oily wheat germ, the reproductive part of the grain. When the germ was crushed during the milling process, its oil spread through the flour, imparting the yellow tinge—and also turning the flour rancid after a few weeks of storage.

Then, in the 1840s, a new milling process that was invented in Hungary succeeded in removing the troublesome wheat germ and its oil. For perhaps the first time in history, housewives now had practical reason to buy white flour. The new product achieved quick popularity because, unlike the older flours—brown or white—it could be stored almost indefinitely without spoiling.

A nutritional price had to be paid for the new flour's better keeping qualities. The discarded wheat germ had been a source of vitamins and minerals, which were now lost to customers who eagerly switched from whole-wheat to white flours. The loss in nutrients was not made up until 1941, when millers began to enrich flour and bread by adding back some of the vitamins and minerals lost in refining. Rice is now similarly enriched, so that the preferred white type is almost as nutritious as unrefined brown.

In the interim, the development of preservatives such as sodium propionate made it possible to retard spoilage caused by the oils that are naturally present in whole-grain breads. Nowadays, consumers can have their choice of either color of bread with reasonable assurance that it is not deficient in any major nutrient.

While affluence encourages people to eat more food, and more processed food, it also helps them avoid the chore of cooking it. Increasingly they eat out. Americans are expected to consume 50 per cent of their meals in restaurants by 1990. About a quarter of all restaurant meals are eaten at fast-food establishments, which cater to a society that is not only mobile but largely occupied outside the home. Most adults,

How family meals have changed —for better and worse

What people eat today is remarkably different from what was eaten at the beginning of the 20th Century, as is indicated at right by graphs of per capita consumption in America of seven classes of food. Only now are scientists beginning to evaluate the impact on health of these trends, which are accelerating all over the world as once-costly foods become widely available.

The big shift over the century has been a sharp rise in meat eating, accompanied by an even sharper fall in consumption of bread, pasta and other grain products. By 1980 Americans were consuming 40 per cent more meat, fish and poultry than in 1910 and only half as much grain.

This change, which has altered the proportions of fiber and fat in the diet, has been linked to increases in heart and artery diseases and in some cancers. Other potentially harmful fats and oils are also increasingly used: Consumption was up 42 per cent. More fatty dairy products were eaten as well (although total poundage in 1980 was little different from that in 1910 because of a shift from whole milk to cheeses, which weigh less).

The dietary changes have many other implications. One reason people grow taller today is apparently the rise in consumption of animal protein. Their teeth may be affected because they eat more sugar. They suffer less from vitamin and mineral deficiencies because they eat more fruit and vegetables, now easily obtainable anywhere in any season at reasonable cost. But they may also put on too much weight because they eat more of everything except grains. Consumption of all other foods has generally risen over the century—although the population changes of World War II and its baby boom created some dramatic if temporary consumption shifts.

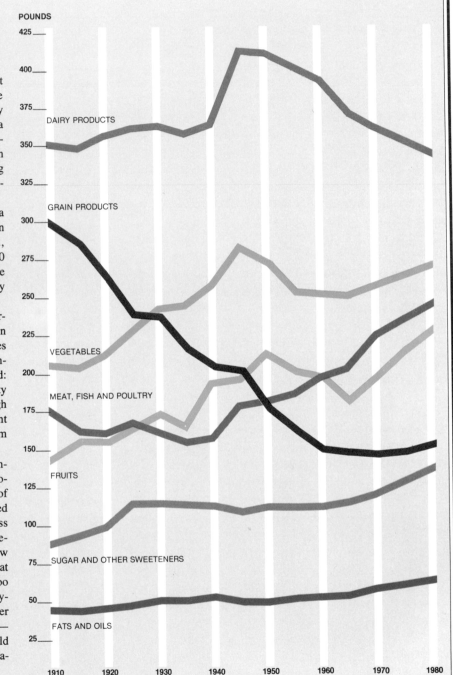

male and female, hold jobs, leaving little time and energy for home cooking. In the United States, about 65 per cent of the mothers of schoolchildren are part of the labor force. Grandmothers, who assumed cooking tasks in the old-fashioned extended family, now live on their own.

The menus of many fast-food restaurants are limited, offering the customer little or no choice of fresh fruits or vegetables, fruit juices or whole-grain breads. Potatoes are almost always deep fried, a fast and convenient cooking process that provides three times the calories, and 130 times the fat, of boiling or baking. Foods are heavily salted, and a beverage such as the typical shake may contain as much as 14 teaspoons of sugar—more than 200 empty calories.

The main dishes served, on the other hand, are surprisingly nutritious, providing a good combination of essential nutrients *(pages 15-17)*. And even the high caloric content of most fast foods may not be excessive for active young people. Commented the nutritionist Jean Mayer, ''Hamburgers, especially those obtained at fast-food restaurants, are high in calories and fat; they are definitely not for dieters. However, if the child is getting fruit, vegetables and milk at other times of the day, hamburgers and similar fast foods can compose part of a balanced diet.''

Meals of mystical power

All the changes brought by the 20th Century have done nothing to alter the basic needs of people. Food must be ample to provide materials for growth and repair of the body and energy for its operation—but not so abundant that excess fat accumulates. Its variety must be balanced so that it protects against disease. The U.S. Department of Agriculture has estimated that changes in diet could reduce the incidence of cancer by 20 per cent, of heart disease by 25 per cent and of diabetes by 50 per cent. But food serves more than the body. It is intimately involved in human behavior, affecting social actions and influencing emotional well-being. So important is food to human culture that the noted French anthropologist Claude Lévi-Strauss traced the nature and development of thought and the rise of civilization to eating habits.

Food serves as a potent medium of communication. It is used to express sympathy or sorrow, to honor personal and professional accomplishments, and to indicate friendliness. ''In some societies,'' wrote anthropologist Dorothy Lee, ''no new relationship can be initiated or no transaction carried on without gifts of food. One man will give to the other a basket of yams and be given a basket of yams in return. The yams are of the same size, kind, and degree of ripeness. The baskets are the same size. All that has happened is that food has been given as a gift, back and forth.''

At times of stress, certain foods assume important roles in relieving tension. During World War II, many U.S. soldiers developed cravings for milk. ''The unhappy, suffering, far-from-home-and-loved-ones soldier,'' wrote psychologist Harriet Bruce Moore, ''looks back to milk as in many ways expressing the comfort, security and contentedness of life as it was at home.'' At the end of the War, the Red Cross greeted GIs returning from the Pacific theater by handing them glasses of milk as they filed off the troopships.

Cultural and religious taboos entangle food. North Americans do not eat termites or grasshoppers, insects that serve as important sources of protein in parts of Africa. India's Hindus do not eat beef. Pork, a staple in much of the West, is shunned by Moslems and Jews. Americans turn pale at the thought of consuming dog meat or horseflesh. Yet in China dog meat has been considered a culinary delicacy since antiquity, and the French have been eating horseflesh since the 18th Century.

In Latin America, many people still choose their foods according to an ancient mythology that ascribes heating and cooling properties to each dish. The origins of this belief are lost in antiquity; the categorizations have no overt connection with either the temperature or the relative spiciness of the food. Thus, fruits, vegetables and pork are classified as cold, while cereals, sugars and some other meats are considered hot. Eating an excess of either hot or cold foods, the Latin Americans believe, can produce illness. Happily, the illness can be cured simply by restoring the proper balance between the two categories.

In China, a somewhat similar classification of food, in this case into the categories yin and yang, has influenced the

Why fast food is not junk food

The hamburgers, pizzas and French fries of fast-food restaurants—perhaps the most popular meals in America and increasingly common in other countries—are often condemned as junk food. Many nutritionists hold a different, and somewhat surprising, opinion. Such foods, they say, balance substantial amounts of nearly all essential nutrients; pizza, for instance, provides protein and fat in its cheese, carbohydrate in its crust, and vitamins and minerals in its tomato sauce. When eaten in normal quantities, the fast foods may supply more calories than the average adult needs—a hamburger, fried potatoes and shake contribute about 1,300 calories, about half the daily adult requirement—but not necessarily more than an active teenager can use.

Unfortunately, fast foods are not entirely free of nutritional drawbacks: Most contain excessive amounts of sodium (principally in salt), sugar and fat. Fat contributes about 50 per cent of the calories in fried fish, chicken and potatoes, and sugar supplies about half of the roughly 300 calories in a 10-ounce shake. The frothy shake also contains about .01 ounce, or 300 milligrams, of sodium; if consumed with, say, half a 10-inch pizza or with a cheeseburger, the sodium intake skyrockets to about .05 ounce, or 1,300 milligrams—as much as an adult needs in a day.

Fast foods are also deficient in fiber and, depending on the foods, in a few vitamins. Folacin, for example, is all but absent in a fast-food meal of hamburger, French fries and shake. No authority recommends fast foods as the sole daily fare. But if the sugary drinks are limited, and if sodium-laced seasonings are shunned, the oft-maligned fast foods meet the ultimate goals of a sound diet: nutritional balance and broad appeal.

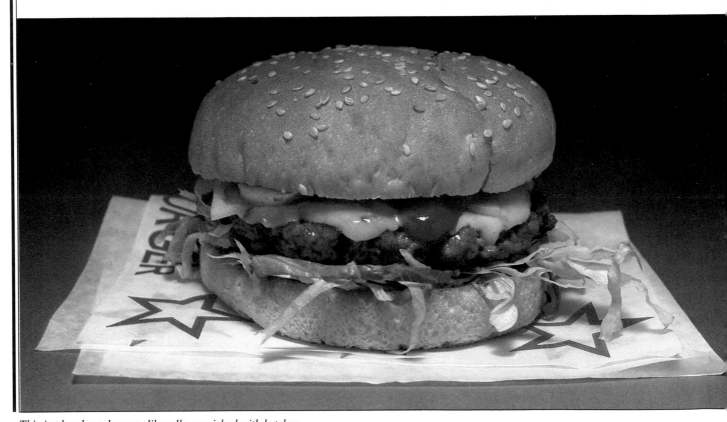

This jumbo cheeseburger, liberally garnished with ketchup, mustard, lettuce and onions, supplies more than 50 per cent of the average adult's daily requirements for protein, vitamin A and niacin, and one third of the recommended amounts of phosphorus and calcium. It also contains 520 calories and approximately an entire day's prudent allotment of fat and sodium.

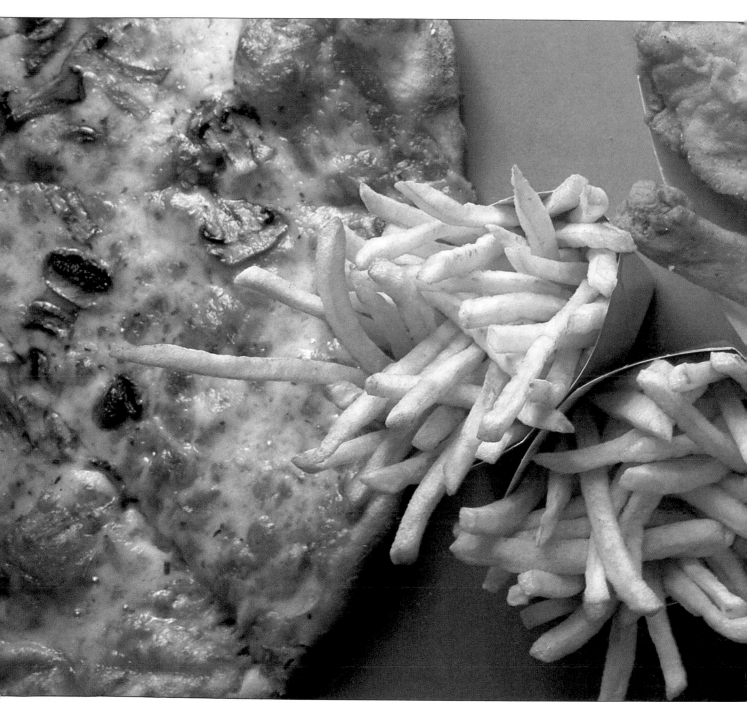

The bubbling cheese that contributes to the 230 calories in a single slice of this 16-inch mushroom pizza also supplies about one third of an adolescent boy's daily protein requirement and some of the calcium essential for his growing bones and teeth. But the slice also contains about .05 ounce, or 1100 milligrams, of sodium—as much as a teen-age boy ought to have in a day.

Each of the six-ounce orders of French fries above is packed with valuable minerals such as potassium, magnesium and phosphorus, and contains significant amounts of nutritious carbohydrates. However, one order adds not only salt but about 550 calories to a meal, nearly half of them from the frying oil that gilds each crisp shoestring with an unwelcome layer of fat.

Three pieces of fried chicken selected from the assortment below will supply approximately 550 calories and roughly 1.5 ounces, or 40 grams, of protein—slightly more than the daily requirement for protein for an adult woman. But, because they are fried, they also contain more than an ounce, or 33 grams, of fat, half the amount recommended in a prudent day's diet.

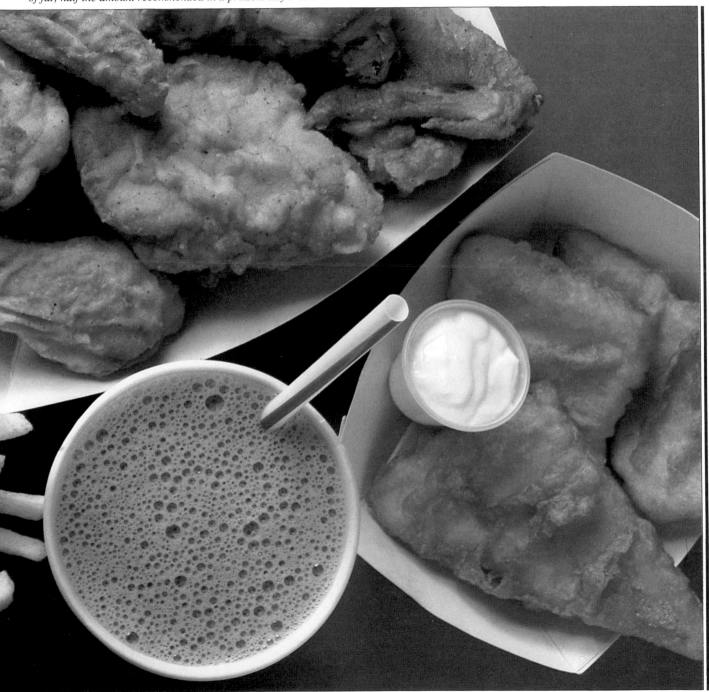

The chocolate shake above contains dried milk, butterfat, sugar, water, artificial flavorings and gum stabilizers whipped up into the nutritional equivalent of a homemade milk shake. Both provide 10 to 50 per cent of a day's supply of magnesium, phosphorus, iron, thiamine, niacin and calcium. This shake's main drawback is its high sodium content and, for adults, its 300 calories.

A typical fast-food serving of fish—two batter-fried fillets of cod—has only two thirds as many calories (about 150 per piece) as other popular main courses. But it contains roughly the same amount of fat and fewer nutrients overall. The serving cup's one-ounce dollop of tartar sauce adds 150 calories and boosts the meal's fat content to an undesirable level.

choice of foods for some 2,500 years. Yang foods, which are considered to have active, masculine attributes, include meats, deep-fried dishes and alcoholic drinks. Yin foods, with feminine and passive qualities, include grains and vegetables. Men are advised not to eat many yang foods, since the attributes of these foods are already predominant in males, while females are likewise warned away from excessive consumption of yin foods.

Similar powers have been ascribed to food in every part of the world. In Persia in the Sixth Century B.C., Cyrus the Great said, "Soft countries give birth to soft men; there was no region that produced very delightful fruits and at the same time men of warlike spirit." In the early 19th Century, the famous British Shakespearean actor Edmund Kean matched his diet to his role; Kean made a practice of eating mutton before he played a lover, pork before a tyrannical part and beef before a murderous one.

Even the brilliant Baron Justus von Liebig thought he had proved that meat provoked ferocity. At a zoo in Giessen, Germany, a bear was fed a diet of bread and vegetables for several days. The researchers duly noted the animal's subsequent gentle nature. Then they fed the bear meat for several days. The caged animal quickly turned vicious. The effects of meat seemed obvious. But Liebig and his colleagues had overlooked the simple fact that a bear confined to a vegetarian diet may have been too weak from undernourishment to attack its gullible keepers.

A banquet of elixirs

Special values continue to be attributed to certain "health foods"—yogurt, honey, bee pollen and ginseng, among many others. Most, including these four, are useful in some way. Whether they achieve as much as their proponents claim remains to be proved.

Yogurt, a fermented milk product, initially acquired its reputation because it is a favored delicacy among peoples of the Caucasus mountains who are famed for their longevity. Repeatedly over the years, reports from this region have told of inhabitants living hale and hearty past the age of 100, their long-lasting vigor attributed to consumption of yogurt. In

fact, few of these yogurt eaters can provide birth certificates or any other proof that they have reached 100 years. According to Zhores A. Medvedev, a Soviet biologist and gerontologist who was exiled to the West in 1973, many old men in the Soviet Caucasus have been fooling observers for years. "The trouble is that many scientists have taken for granted that these old people are telling the truth," said Medvedev, "and then they try to find some reasons to explain their supposed longevity."

Medvedev pointed to the value of exaggerating age in the Soviet Union. The elderly receive increasing honor and respect as they age and are often venerated as "a special social achievement of the Soviet Union." In addition, Caucasus longevity drew the enthusiastic attention of Soviet dictator Josef Stalin, who came from that region. Local authorities felt compelled to look for local centenarians to support Stalin's belief in the virtues of his homeland. But mainly, Medvedev suggests, the supposedly aged men were draft dodgers or deserters who obtained false papers during World War I and several years of subsequent civil war. There was one man who claimed to be 128 years old until fellow villagers recognized him as their 78-year-old former neighbor. The fake centenarian, a deserter from the Army during World War I, had adopted his father's identification papers to make himself overage for the military. Yogurt had not increased his life span—or anyone else's.

Less spectacular claims are made for other health foods such as honey and bee pollen, but these claims too may be overstated. Many people have a belief that honey, the natural sweetener produced by bees from plant nectar, is somehow more nutritious than table sugar is, even though honey contains approximately the same number of calories, the same amounts of vitamins, and only negligibly larger amounts of such minerals as calcium, potassium and phosphorus. Some health-food stores promote organic honey, which is supposedly free of pesticides and insecticides—even though in fact it is virtually impossible, in most parts of the world, to find plants growing in soil that is completely free of these kinds of substances.

While making their nectar-collecting rounds, bees also

accumulate quantities of pollen, the microscopic grains containing the male reproductive element of flowering plants. For hundreds of years, people have collected this pollen from beehives. The product, known as bee pollen, is now sold as a preparation that confers great athletic prowess on its users. Although bee pollen can be a nutritious source of protein and vitamins, a study at Louisiana State University failed to uncover any other useful properties. A group of the university's athletes who took 10 tablets of bee pollen per day for six weeks showed no improvement in performance over their colleagues who had taken neutral dummy pills for the same span of time.

Some claims made for health foods have been verified. In China and other Oriental countries, the root of the ginseng plant has been prized for centuries as a cure for numerous diseases and as a potent aphrodisiac. Ginseng's qualities as a love potion and panacea are still to be proved, but medical researchers in the U.S.S.R. and the Far East have reported that teas brewed from it do relieve tension and the digestive disorders often associated with stress.

In order to enjoy whatever beneficial properties ginseng may possess, however, the consumer also has to risk certain less desirable side effects. Like a few other herbs used for tea, it contains minute quantities of several toxic chemicals. "Among its toxic effects," said Dr. Victor Herbert, at the Downstate Medical Center of the State University of New York, "are diarrhea, skin eruptions, insomnia, nervousness and severe mental confusion."

Few health foods are likely to cause harm. Because the majority are traditional favorites, their safety is generally attested to by centuries of use. However, they generally are costlier than less exotic products sold in regular supermarkets, and their special values remain to be accepted by medical authorities.

You can make up a wholesome diet more simply. Just choose a balance of foods that are appealing to your individual taste from among vegetables and fruits, breads and cereals, milk and cheese, and meat, poultry, fish and beans—and eat no more of these foods than you need to maintain your weight at a desirable level. ❋

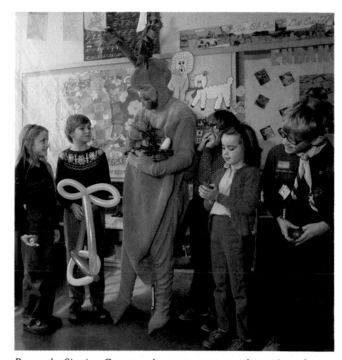

Roger the Singing Carrot—the orange-costumed creation of actor Bill Wood—serenades five Maine schoolchildren with a doleful ballad about the cold, lonely life of an uneaten vegetable. Wood's one-man show, sponsored jointly by the University of Maine and a local community action group, emphasizes the importance of eating healthful, well-balanced meals.

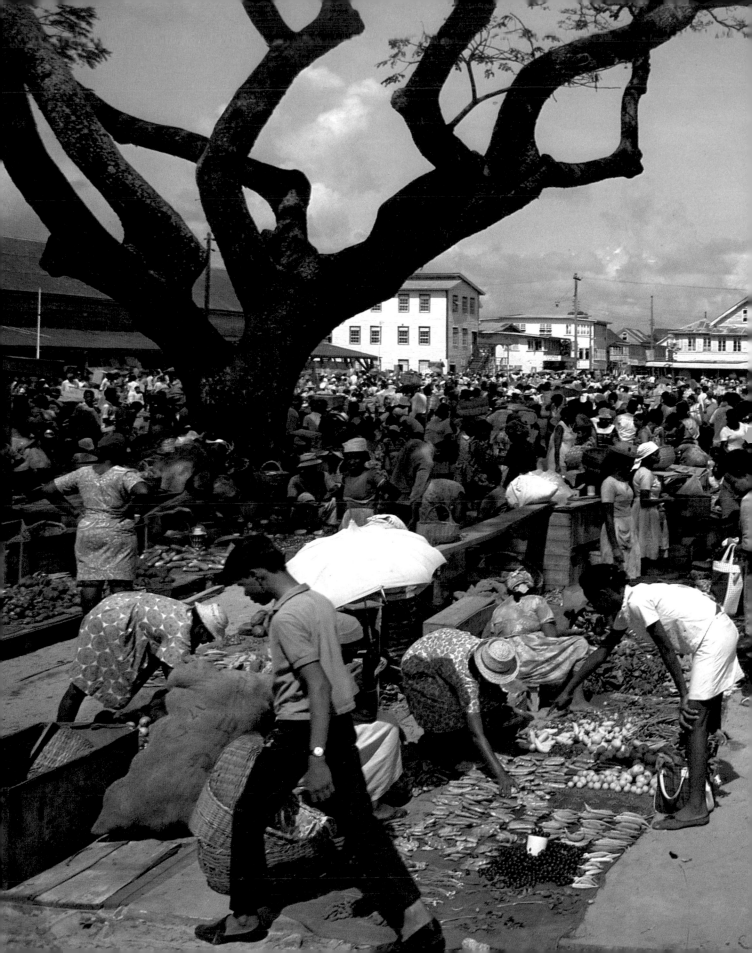

Diverse diets that nourish the world

For centuries people of different lands have incorporated their foods—and the nutrients they contain—into distinctive traditional diets. From a nutritional standpoint, almost every ethnic diet—six are represented on these and the following pages—supplies enough of the more than 40 nutrients that a human being needs to grow up healthy and stay that way. Each diet is built around grain: corn in Mexico, for example, rice in Japan, rye and wheat in Russia. Additional nutrients are derived from whatever fruits, vegetables and animal products the land affords.

Although most traditional menus are adequate, none makes for a perfect diet. The Russian diet is rich in fats, linked to heart disease; the Japanese in salt, a cause of hypertension. As for the Italians, they have a perfectly sound diet; they simply enjoy their foods too much and have a national weight problem to show for it.

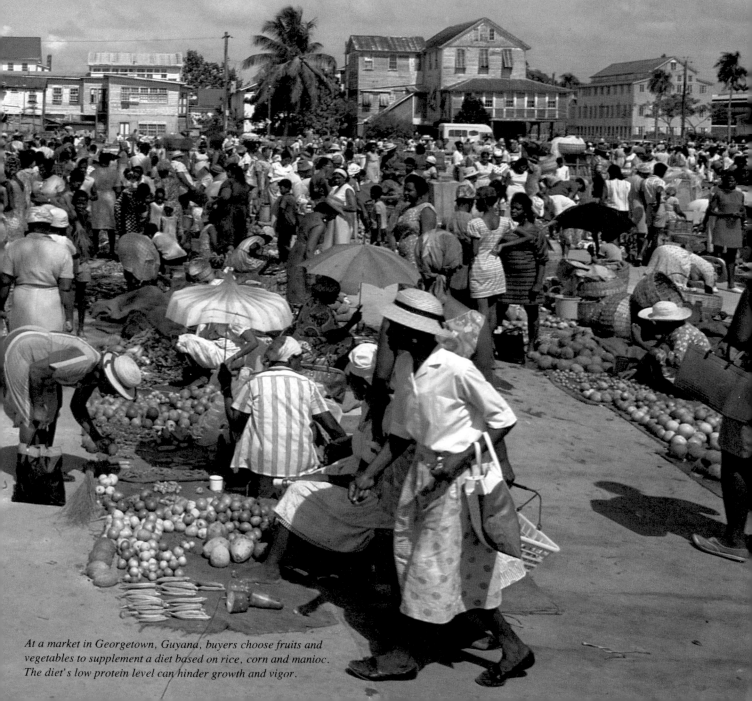

At a market in Georgetown, Guyana, buyers choose fruits and vegetables to supplement a diet based on rice, corn and manioc. The diet's low protein level can hinder growth and vigor.

Italy: the power of pasta

The Italian diet, known for breads and rice dishes as well as for pastas, is one of the world's best-balanced. A typical daily ration of bread and pasta—about three fourths of a pound—supplies ample carbohydrate and about 40 per cent of the day's protein, a figure nutritionists consider desirable because such protein lacks the fat found in meat and dairy products. The average Italian also consumes more than a half pound of fruit and a pound of vegetables daily, ensuring sufficient vitamins, minerals and fiber.

Supplementing this healthful menu are fats and additional proteins in the light forms believed to lessen the chance of heart disease—olive oil, and lean meats such as veal and poultry. Indeed, Italians enjoy a low rate of coronary heart disease. But their enthusiastic wine consumption brings on liver disease, and as a group they take in 30 per cent more calories than they need.

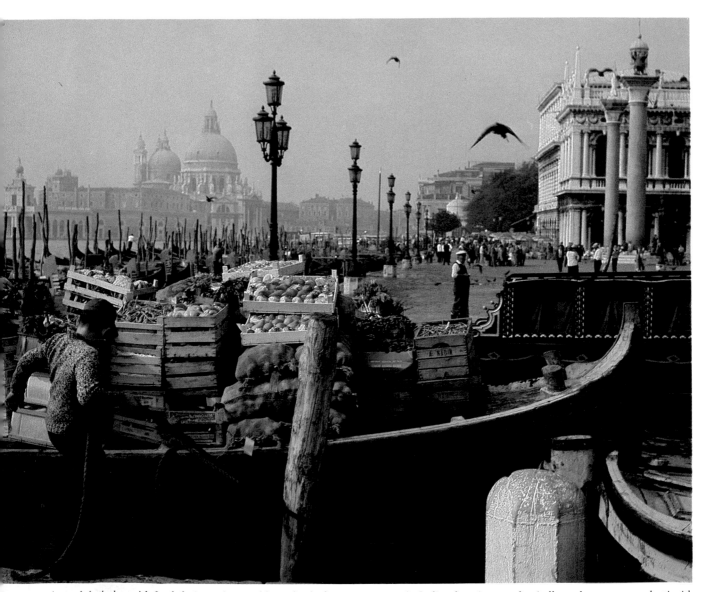

A gondola laden with fresh fruits and vegetables—foods that add vitamins and minerals to the pasta-based Italian diet—makes a stop in a Venetian canal. The tomatoes (left), used in zesty sauces for pasta, are a good source of vitamin C; the leafy greens, consumed in salads, provide such minerals as magnesium and iron, good for building bones and red blood cells.

An Italian favorite, spaghetti alla carbonara—spaghetti with eggs, prosciutto ham and cheese—fills a plate on a picturesque balcony. The spaghetti, made from a hard spring wheat called durum, is approximately 13 per cent protein by weight; the animal products that garnish the pasta increase the amount of protein in the meal—but also increase the amount of fat.

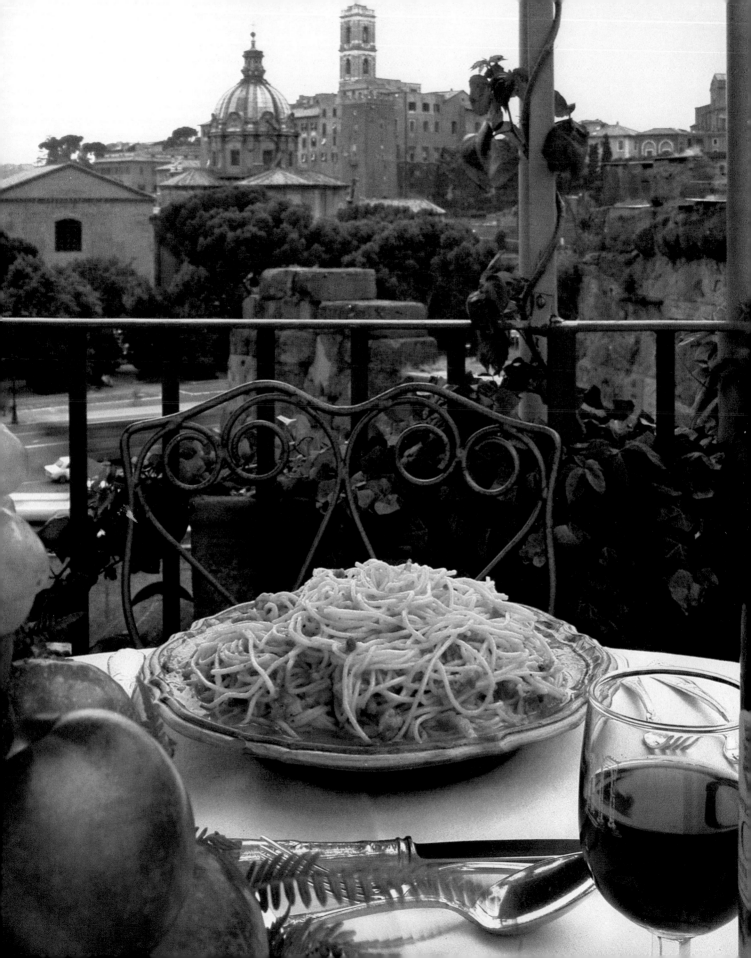

Japan: mixed blessings of rice and fish

A Japanese meal simply would not be Japanese without rice. Served for lunch, dinner and even breakfast, rice provides nearly two thirds of the average person's daily carbohydrates, almost a third of his protein and more than half of his total calories.

Rice is nourishing, but the Japanese prefer it polished, made white and less bulky by a process that strips away the bran layer, where fiber and many key nutrients are stored. Such rice retains only one third of its niacin, one fifth of its thiamine and three fifths of its riboflavin—vitamins that help the body use food energy. It also retains little fiber, believed important in cancer prevention.

More damaging, though, are the salty foods eaten with rice: soy sauce and salted fish. Authorities believe such a diet may alter the stomach wall, promoting cancer *(page 104)*; the Japanese lead the world in the incidence of stomach cancer.

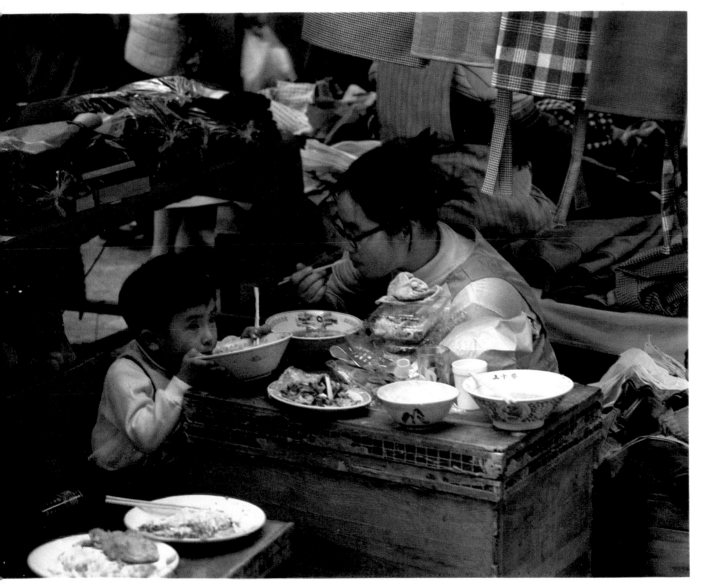

In the family tailor shop, a Japanese mother and son break for a midday meal that includes the traditional polished rice plus a noodle broth and assorted vegetables. The meal contains ample nutrients—although there is no meat, the soybean products in the broth offer a supply of protein.

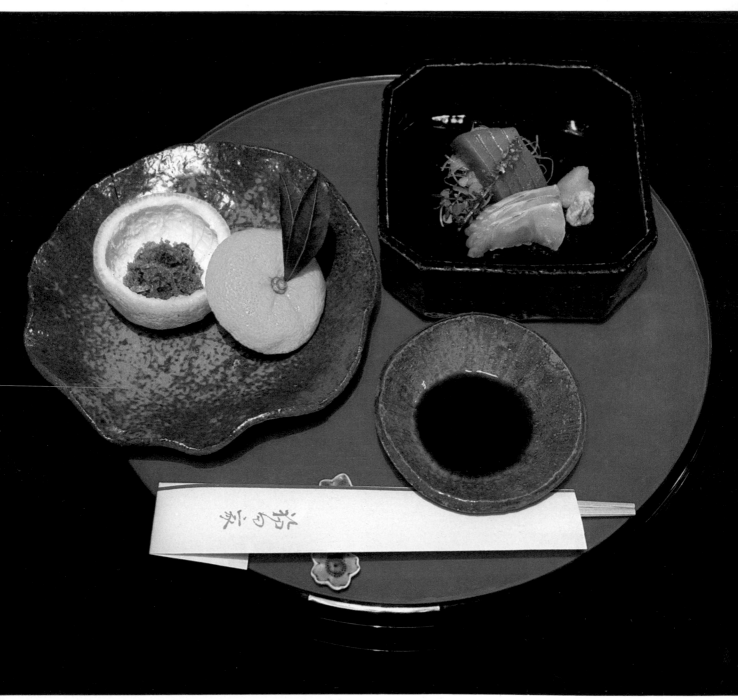

Japanese delicacies—sliced seafood and roe in lemon (above, left), raw fish with condiments (top), and salty soy sauce—create an appealing plate. This traditional dish is typically low in fat; the Japanese derive a mere 12.6 per cent of their calories from fat, perhaps explaining their low rate of heart disease.

Mexico: a happy marriage of corn and beans

The cornerstone of Mexico's diet is the versatile grain, corn, which was domesticated there around 3000 B.C. It can be prepared in various ways, but in most Mexican meals it takes the shape of the tortilla, a pancake made from ground cornmeal.

Yet Mexicans do not—indeed, could not—live by corn and tortilla alone; doing so would leave them without essential components of protein. In practice, Mexicans couple their corn dishes with frijoles, or beans—which also lack a protein component but are rich in those that corn does not provide. When beans and corn are eaten at the same meal, the result is a "complete" protein, one that, like those in meat, contains all the ingredients humans need. The solution is not a perfect one: If the foods are eaten even a few hours apart, the combination effect is lost, and Mexican authorities consider protein sufficiency their country's key dietary goal.

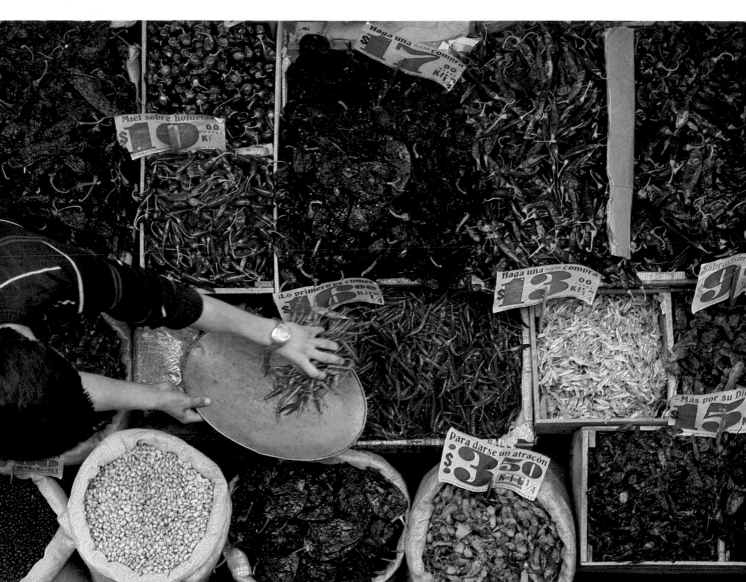

A Mexican woman selects a handful of dried chili peppers from a market display that also includes beans (bottom left) and dried fruit (bottom, second from right). The peppers' fiery taste, derived from a chemical called capsaicin, might seem to make this food harmful. It is not. Indeed, chilies supply more vitamin A than most plants, as well as vitamin C and several B vitamins.

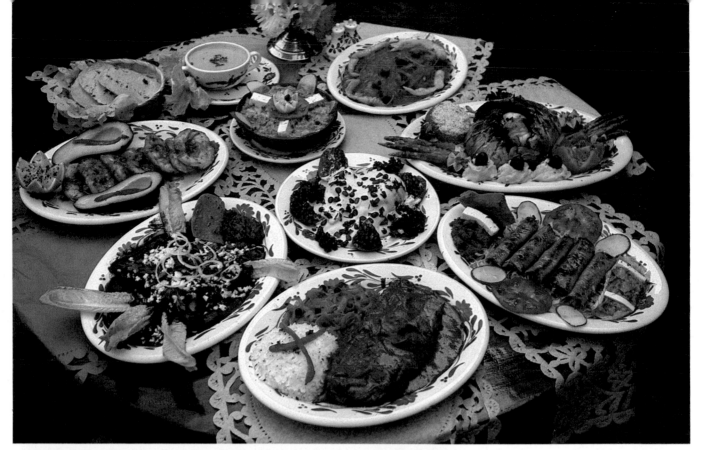

An inviting array of Mexican specialties—
more lavish and certainly higher in fat
than an average meal—adorns a banquet
table. Clockwise from top are liberally
garnished plates of red snapper, lobster
tails, chicken tacos with refried beans,
steamed chicken, enchiladas (rolled tortillas
stuffed with meat), grilled shrimp and
squash-flower soup. At center are peppers
stuffed with beef and guacamole, made
with mashed avocados.

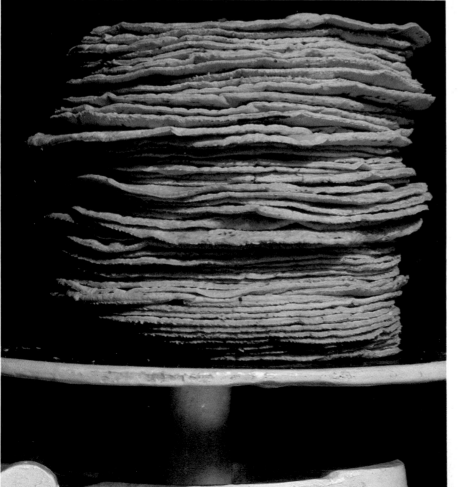

Paper-thin tortillas form an impressive stack
on a market scale. The dried corn that is
used to make meal for tortillas is soaked in
limewater, a calcium hydroxide solution;
the grain's calcium content is thus multiplied
20 times and the ground flour provides
the body with the mineral it most needs to
build and maintain the bones and teeth.

Russia: varied grains, dairy riches

In the Ukraine and throughout the Soviet Union, grain products are the staple of the diet. What distinguishes the Ukrainian diet, however, is its variety of grains: Rye and wheat are turned into breads, and buckwheat is made into a coarse meal called *kasha*. The variety of grains helps balance their differing protein ingredients, and *kasha* is normally cooked with eggs or onions, mushrooms, soup stock, chicken or meat—a practice that rounds it out with animal proteins and fats and produces a nourishing dish.

Much of the fat Russians consume—as in sour cream for *borshch (right)* and butter for *bliny (below)*—is the saturated type linked to heart disease. In the past, such foods were eaten in amounts that apparently caused little harm. But after World War II, more foods high in saturated fat began to reach Russian tables, contributing to a heart disease rate that doubled in 20 years.

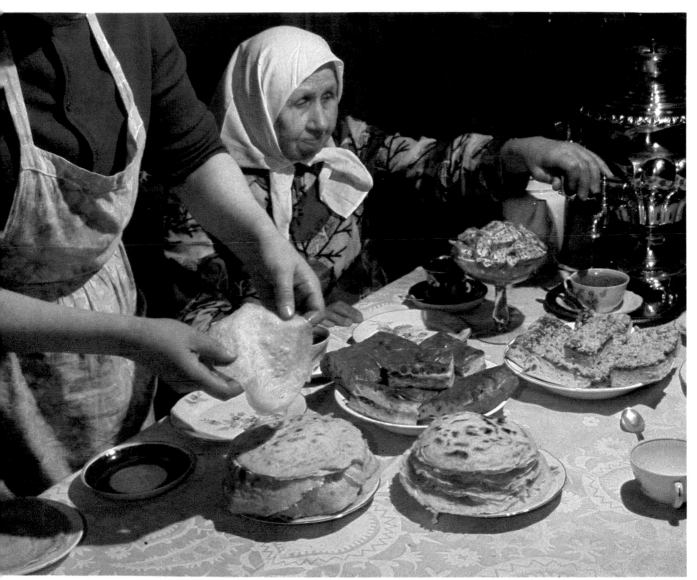

A Russian grandmother pours tea from a traditional samovar while her daughter serves bliny from a stack of the delectable pancakes. Made from buckwheat flour and yeast, bliny are quite nutritious by themselves. But Russian custom is to slather them with anything from salmon and herring to sour cream and butter, loading them with extra calories and dangerous fat.

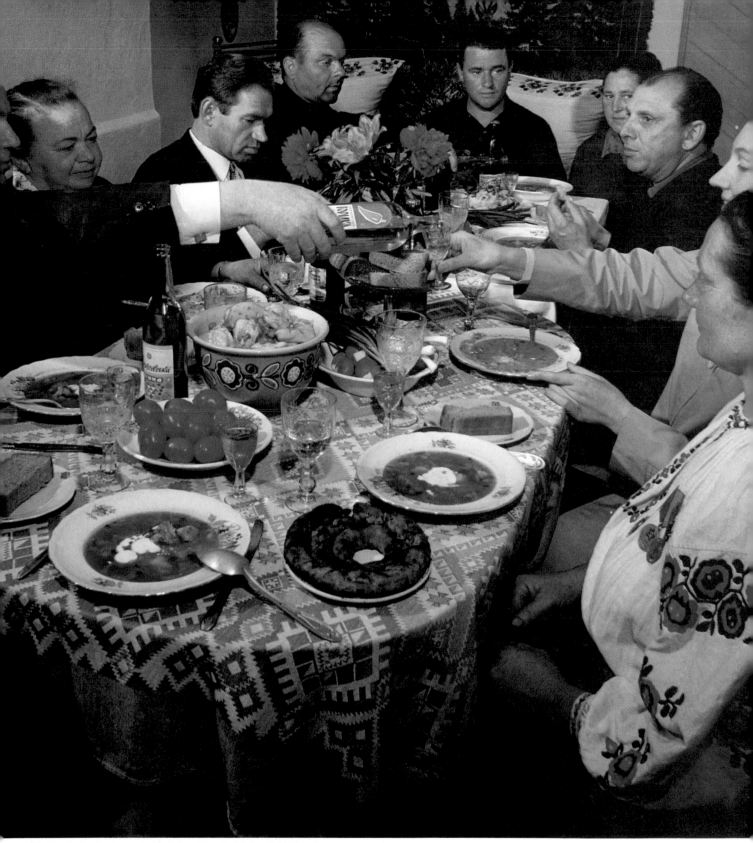

Vodka flows freely at a Ukrainian dinner celebration that features the traditional beet soup called borshch, served with sour cream, and varenyky, the meat-filled dumplings in the large bowl. With its numerous side dishes, the meal is nutritionally complete; but it almost surely offers more fat and calories than the average Ukrainian needs — including those in the vodka.

Greece: a Mediterranean harvest

Thanks partly to a mild and maritime location, Greeks are able to fill out a menu based on bread with the abundant and nutritious fruit of their land and of the sea. Lemons, oranges, grapes, peaches, berries, melons and figs provide vitamins and minerals, as do vegetables such as onions, tomatoes and zucchini. Fish is a popular protein source, supplemented by the Greeks' favorite meat, lamb. Unlike most fish, but like other red meats, lamb contains fats considered harmful. Yet, partly because it is expensive and partly because cooking fuel for roasting is either expensive or scarce, the meat is eaten only once or twice a week.

What sets the Greek diet apart from much of the world's, however, is the kind of fat consumed in quantity: olive oil. It contains little of the saturated fats that are present in meats, butter and most shortenings used for cooking in Northern Europe and America.

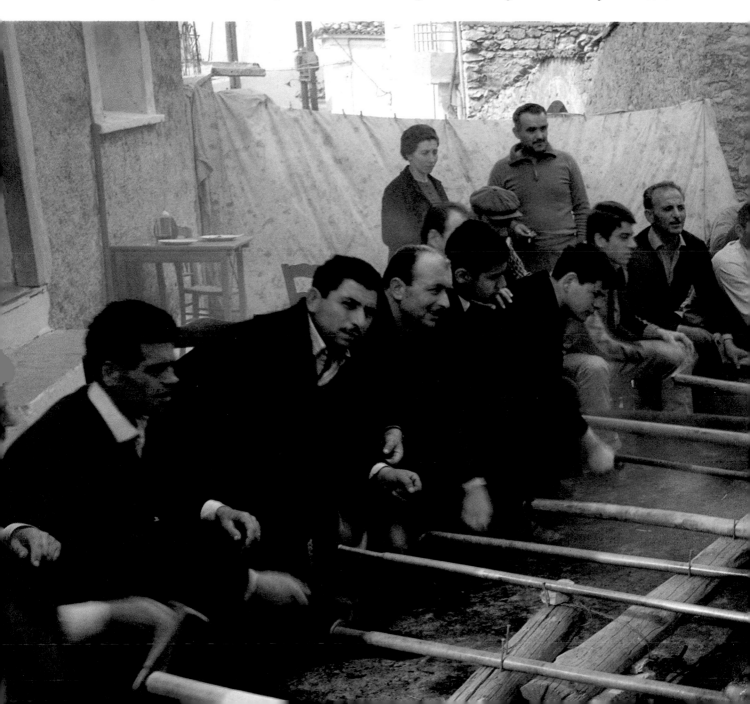

31

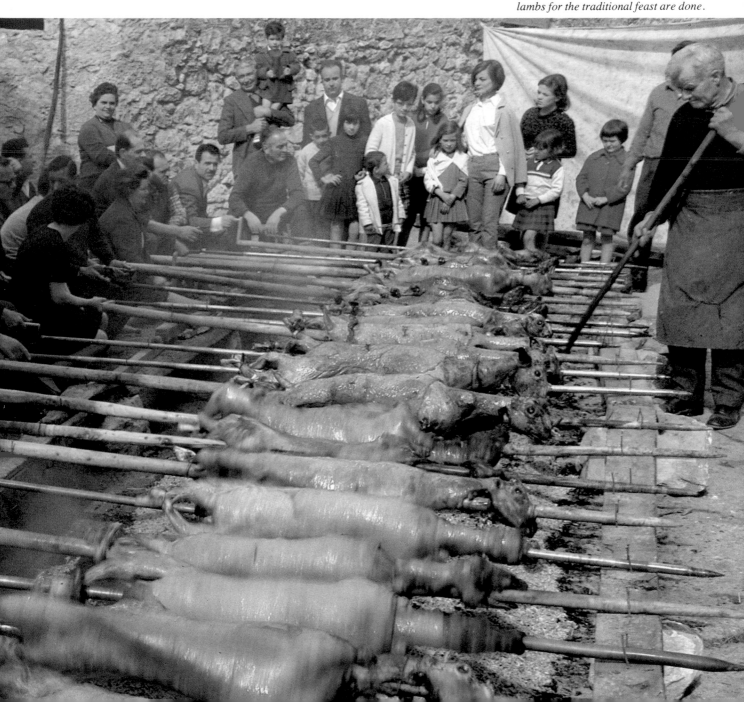

Early on Easter morning, the villagers of Delphi gather at their communal roasting pit to rotate the spits until the paschal lambs for the traditional feast are done.

What food is made of

A loaf of bread, a jug of wine, etc., may have guaranteed bliss for the 11th Century poet-mathematician Omar the Tentmaker. But it falls short of what is now known to be necessary to keep your body and soul together.

At least 25 different chemical elements, from calcium to zinc, are needed to make up the human body. With the exception of a few that you breathe in air, they all come from the ingredients of food, most in the form of complex chemical compounds that have to be broken down and reassembled to fulfill their functions. To keep your body in repair and to power its operation, the proper variety and amounts of these ingredients must be available in the foods you eat.

Once inside the body, food undergoes a transmutation in the process called metabolism. The basic components of food, lifeless chemicals, are changed into living cells, tissues, organs. They build new bone, muscle and blood, and replace or replenish body parts that have been damaged, worn out or sloughed off. Hair, nails and skin are obvious examples of tissues that are constantly being replaced. The inner lining of the intestine is a less obvious one: It is changed every three or four days. About a quarter of the red blood cells must be replaced every month. The connective tissue called collagen is turned over about once every 10 years.

Building and maintaining body parts is not enough. Metabolism also generates energy. Some of the energy provides heat to maintain the body at a high enough temperature; below a certain point, it would simply stop operating. Food energy also enables the body to conduct all the myriad electrochemical processes essential to life and, beyond that, to do external work. At perfect rest, in profound slumber, you require a substantial amount of energy. But to move, work or play you need a good deal more.

Scientists calculate the energy content of food in units that are confusingly called calories but are a thousand times larger than the calories defined in school science texts; one food calorie is the amount of heat energy required to raise the temperature of a liter (about one quart) of water 1° C. (1.8° F.). Researchers can determine the calorie content of any food by burning it in a device called a calorimeter and then measuring the amount of heat produced—a process roughly analogous to what happens in the body. (The technique for this measurement was invented by one of the more notable victims of the French Revolution's guillotine, the chemist Antoine-Laurent Lavoisier, who had the misfortune to be an investor in the hated office of tax collector.)

A hamburger has 235 calories. By contrast, a gallon of gasoline has 30,432. Between the ages of 20 and 70, an average adult will consume about 36 million calories. About 60 per cent of this energy will sustain the metabolism. The rest, if not consumed in other ways, would result in a weight gain of two tons of fat.

It is possible—for a time—to acquire materials that power and build the body from a very restricted diet. In 1910, reported M. Hindhede of the Laboratory of Nutritional Experimentation in Copenhagen, a Danish investigator remained hale, if not hearty, for a year on nothing but potatoes.

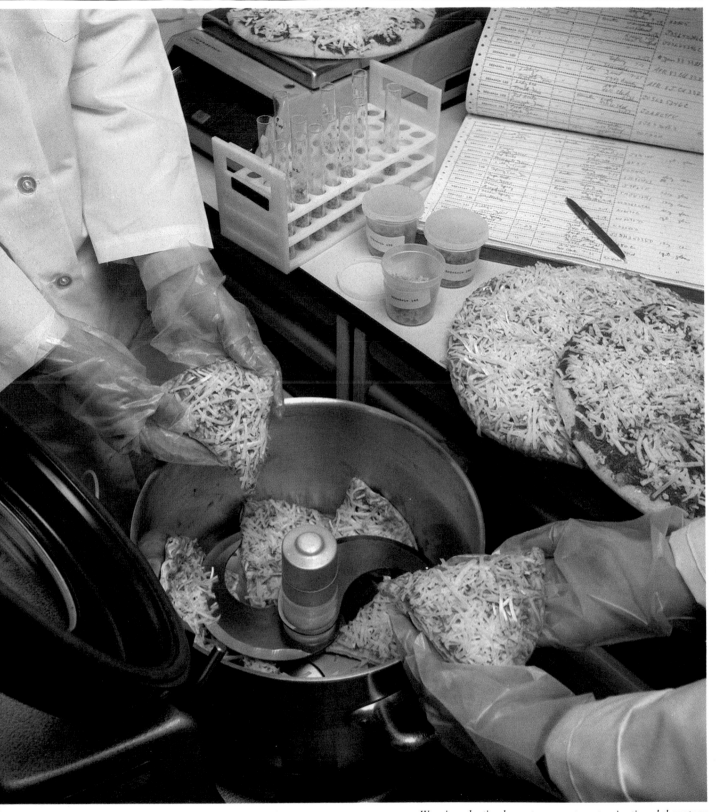

Wearing plastic gloves to prevent contamination, laboratory technicians drop slices of preweighed, store-bought frozen pizza into a four-gallon industrial blender—the first step in an analysis of the nutritional value of this popular food. Within seconds the blender reduces the pizza to a homogeneous, doughy mush that can be placed in test tubes and lab dishes for study.

Angus Barbieri, in the process of reducing from 472 pounds to 178 in Maryfield Hospital, Dundee, Scotland, in 1965 and 1966, went without solid food for 13 months, subsisting on only tea, coffee, soda water and vitamins. Such feats are possible, most authorities believe, only when reserves of essential ingredients from other foods are already stored in the body to be drawn upon. Their presence makes up for the deficiencies in the severely limited diets.

Most people consume an assortment of foods. The variety of plants and animals eaten around the world is incredibly diverse, ranging from plums to periwinkles. But geography and economics put many foods beyond the reach of large groups of people. And subtle cultural differences between one heritage and another dictate that dog, monkey and guinea pig shall be acceptable among some peoples but not among others, that snakes and grubs shall be considered delicacies among Australian aborigines but not among Parisians, and that all meats are abhorrent to some Hindus and Buddhists.

Almost any prolonged limitation of diet, however it arises, affects health. The basic materials needed to provide energy and substance for the body—nutrients—are so numerous, and the requirements so changeable, that omitting a single food type may deprive the body of something it needs. Too much is just as bad. Reliance on one or a few kinds of foods may introduce a harmful excess of materials that, in smaller quantities, are necessary.

A mix of 40 ingredients—plus water

How much of what foods is enough—and not too much—is a question that continues to be debated. The ideal diet remains elusive. But there is now general agreement on the basic materials that are needed to keep most people healthy. One of the great triumphs of modern medicine has been the isolation of more than 40 chemical elements and specific compounds essential to human health. Most of these nutrients have been traced to their destinations in the body, so that the reason they are needed is understood. And the amounts required have been gauged with enough precision so that scientists can recommend daily allotments that will keep most people in good health.

Nutrients are divided according to their chemical composition and their biological roles into three main groups of macronutrients: carbohydrates, fats and proteins. These, along with water, make up the bulk of food. Present with the macronutrients in small quantities—and thus called micronutrients—are vitamins and minerals. Some of the macro- and micronutrients can be manufactured by the body's own chemical processing plant from other ingredients—fats can be made from carbohydrates, for example. But others cannot be synthesized within the body; these "essential" nutrients must be obtained directly from food. Some vitamins and minerals are essential nutrients: Vitamin K can be manufactured by the digestive system, but vitamin C must be present ready-made in food.

Of the substances needed in large quantities, one simple, common compound is not ordinarily counted as a nutrient, although it is the most important: water. Its absence will bring death faster than the lack of any other component of the diet. Even two to three days without water may be fatal. The longest documented survival without water (and food) was achieved in 1977 by a remarkable 19-year-old Rumanian, Sorin Crainic, who was entombed under rubble in Bucharest for 10½ days after an earthquake.

There is more water in the human body than anything else. It makes up about two thirds of the average adult's total weight. Blood is 80 per cent water, bone about 25 per cent. Water not only serves as a transport medium, carrying nutrients, waste products and the body's own chemical regulators and disease fighters where they are needed; it also acts as lubricant and solvent to keep the machinery of the body running properly.

Between two and three quarts of water are consumed each day to replace the amount typically lost in perspiration, urine, feces and exhaled breath. Much more is needed by people who exercise in hot weather. Insufficient water causes not only acute thirst but also potentially dangerous changes in body metabolism, including a rise in temperature. Too much water in hot weather, when perspiration removes it from the system quickly, carries away soluble minerals the body must have; unless extra salt is taken with the water the result can be

A big box for counting calories

Around the turn of the century at Wesleyan University in Middletown, Connecticut, it was not unusual for students of Professor Wilbur O. Atwater to climb into a large, airtight copper box *(below)* and stay there for 10 days, sleeping on a tiny folding bed, exercising on a stationary bicycle, taking in carefully measured portions of food through a small window and handing out bodily wastes. With that big box, Atwater, a Wesleyan chemistry professor who was also chief of nutritional experiments for the U.S. Department of Agriculture, was making the first accurate determination of human metabolism, learning how the body uses oxygen to burn up its food the way a furnace burns up fuel.

The sealed copper box, called a respiration calorimeter, was equipped with a ventilation system that blew in fresh air and extracted used air. Instruments measured waste products—water vapor and carbon dioxide—in the used air, and an elaborate scheme detected heat thrown off by the subject. Pipes inside the chamber's walls circulated chilled water, its temperature measured to the hundredth of a degree as it entered the calorimeter and again as it left; because all energy eventually becomes heat, the difference in temperatures corresponded to the amount of energy that the subject generated from the food he ate.

Atwater discovered that during deep sleep the human body burns 60 to 75 food calories per hour; while sitting quietly it burns 100 to 115; and while pedaling a stationary bicycle 300 to 600 calories per hour. His work established direct relationships between activity and the body's use of food that have enabled nutritionists to specify the types of meals and numbers of calories people require to maintain—or reduce to—a healthy weight.

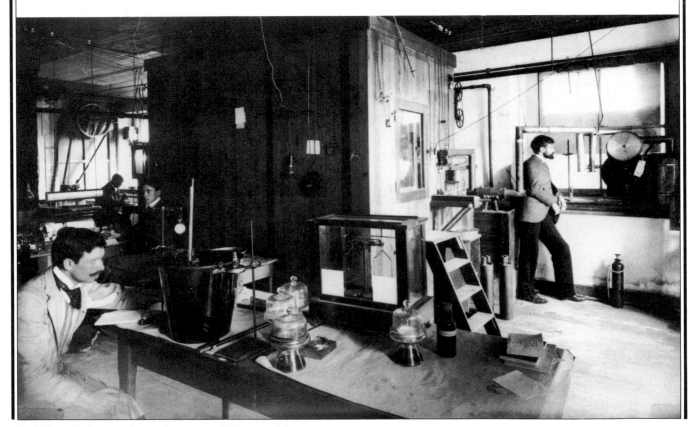

Sealed inside the large box in the center of this turn-of-the-century photograph is a volunteer taking part in the pioneering measurements of human metabolism conducted by Wilbur O. Atwater of Wesleyan University. Four associates monitor gauges and record data to determine the energy produced by the subject from his food—a way of establishing his caloric needs.

a drop in blood pressure, weakness and cramps. Some water is consumed as such, but about half comes from food, which contains astonishingly large amounts: Lettuce is 96 per cent water, eggs 75 per cent, and white bread about 30 per cent.

Taken together, the foods making up most people's meals provide not only water but also all three of the macronutrients, although in varying proportions. For example, lettuce is mostly carbohydrates, bread is largely carbohydrates with some proteins, while eggs are a rich mixture of proteins and fats. Each of the three macronutrients is a distinctive type of chemical compound.

Although all three are necessary for health, carbohydrates stand out because in all but the richest societies they are the staff of life. Carbohydrates make up 65 per cent of the average diet worldwide; even in Canada, the United States and Western Europe they account for almost half the diet. They are a principal source of energy for life. Each ounce of carbohydrates burned in the body engine yields 120 calories. Carbohydrates also add flavor to foods, provide some vitamins and are themselves incorporated into tissue, although they make up a very small part of the body compared to other nutrients. A young man weighing 143 pounds totes around roughly 88 pounds of water, 24 of proteins, 20 of fats and nine of minerals, but only two pounds of carbohydrates.

Carbohydrates are chemical compounds classed as either fibers, sugars or starches. They consist of carbon, hydrogen and oxygen: With a few exceptions, each molecule of carbohydrate always contains twice as many hydrogen atoms as oxygen atoms. The more carbon atoms a carbohydrate molecule contains, the more complex it is considered by food chemists. The simple sugars, such as fructose (found in fruit) and glucose (found in honey and grape juice), are molecules

with only six carbon atoms each. The double sugars, such as sucrose (table sugar), are essentially combinations of two simple sugars and contain 12 carbon atoms each. More complex still, containing as many as 180,000 carbon atoms per molecule, are the starches. One type of complex carbohydrates, fiber such as cellulose, is indigestible by humans although it supports all grazing animals and plays a useful role in human nutrition, providing the roughage and bulk that help the digestive tract eliminate wastes.

Most carbohydrates come from plant foods, principally cereal grains: rice, corn, wheat, oats, barley and millet. They are abundant as well in potatoes, peas, beans, cassava, taro, all fruits, sugar cane and sugar beets. Many processed foods are loaded with carbohydrates, including the starches of pastas, breads and other baked goods as well as the sugars in candies, jams, soft drinks, cakes and even condiments such as ketchup.

Not all foods contain the same kinds of carbohydrates, and the type—simple or complex—is important. Foods such as candy and soft drinks, containing the simple type—sugars—produce energy almost instantly. They are very dense in calories, and if consumed in any quantity provide more energy than the body can burn up. The excess energy converts carbohydrates into fat, adding weight that may be undesirable. Sugars are also a factor in tooth decay (Chapter 4).

The complex carbohydrates—starches such as whole grains, potatoes and pastas—are less rich in calories. Although widely shunned because of the myth that they are fattening, they are less likely to add unwanted weight than the simpler carbohydrates. Because the complex carbohydrate foods contain much water and indigestible fiber, they are much more filling than candy or cake; thus they are much

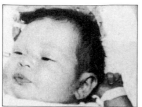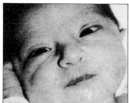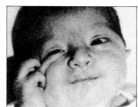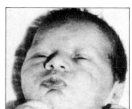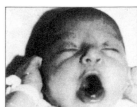

Less than 20 hours old, a baby in an Israeli study confirms that the human preference for sweets is present at birth. From left to right, the baby first rests expressionless without stimulus, next indicates mild satisfaction after a taste of water, then responds to a sugar solution with a pleased smile—but purses his lips at a sour taste and, finally, seems to reject bitter quinine water.

less likely to be eaten in fattening excess. In addition, they provide vitamins, minerals and in some cases protein—all largely missing from the sugars.

Unfortunately, human beings are born with a sweet tooth; tests on babies immediately after birth, before they have had their first taste of milk, indicate that a preference for sugars is innate *(left)*. The human sweet tooth is indulged around the world wherever economic conditions permit. In Great Britain, per capita sugar consumption averages approximately 95 pounds per year; in the United States it is more than 90 pounds per year. And as standards of living go up, so does the consumption of sugar: Sugars accounted for less than one third of the carbohydrates eaten by Americans just before World War I; a half century later the proportion had risen to more than one half.

Even richer in calories than carbohydrates—and thus more likely to cause unwanted weight gain—are foods containing the group of macronutrients called fats. When fats are processed in the body, they generate more than twice as much energy as carbohydrates; the extra energy may not be used up, becoming extra weight. Fats are also implicated in diseases of the heart and blood vessels. Yet fats serve a useful function beyond providing energy. In the body, fat cushions organs such as the kidneys, forms an energy storage depot under the skin and keeps heat from escaping too fast. Fats carry vitamins A, D, E and K. One part of fat, linoleic acid, is an essential nutrient: It cannot be manufactured by the body, and is vital for normal growth and healthy skin. Fortunately, it is present in adequate amounts in many kinds of foods and is abundant in vegetable oils, some nuts and poultry. Fats slow digestion and contribute to the pleasant feeling of fullness that wards off the next round of hunger pangs. And finally, fats make many foods taste good.

Understanding the role of fats in the human diet, and particularly the debate over the part these substances play in heart and blood-vessel disease, is made more difficult by the fact that fats are relatively complicated compounds. They are made up of two types of chemicals: an alcohol named glycerol plus three of the so-called fatty acids. The fatty acids endow each food fat with its unique qualities of flavor and texture, making olive oil quite different from, say, bacon fat.

Each fatty-acid molecule has atoms of hydrogen and oxygen linked to a spine of carbon atoms. The length of the spine varies in edible fats from four to 20 or so carbon atoms. When every carbon atom in the string is linked to as many hydrogen atoms as it can hold, the fatty acid is called saturated. If there are enough spaces in the molecule to hang on two additional hydrogen atoms, it is called monounsaturated. And if there are enough empty places to accommodate four or more hydrogen atoms, the fatty acid is called polyunsaturated. These categories also apply to the fats containing the specific fatty acid; thus the label on a jar of peanut butter may list the amounts of saturated fat and polyunsaturated fat. The saturated fats get most of the blame for damage to the blood system, and monounsaturated fats are believed to cause less harm. Polyunsaturated fats may help protect against circulatory ailments—but all fats have been implicated in cancer.

All dietary fats have some combination of saturated and unsaturated fatty acids, but the ratio depends mainly on whether the fat is of animal or vegetable origin. Foods from animal sources, such as meat, butter, milk, cheese and eggs, are high in saturated fats, which are usually solid at room temperature. Vegetable oils, on the other hand, such as corn oil, sunflower oil and sesame oil, are high in polyunsaturated fats, which are generally liquid at room temperature. Peanut oil and olive oil, also liquids, are high in monounsaturated fats.

There are exceptions, however, making it tricky to tailor a diet to avoid saturated fats. Chocolate, a plant product, is very rich in saturated fats. And palm and coconut oils, both liquids from plants, are among the most highly saturated of all known fats. Few coffee drinkers who buy nondairy creamers to avoid the saturated fats in real cream are aware that the nondairy products are even more saturated because they contain coconut oil.

Reducing fat consumption is further complicated by the fact that although many sources of food fats are obvious, some are not. Nuts, fish and poultry all contain fats: Pecans are 70 to 80 per cent fat. Similarly rich in fats are many processed foods, including baked goods such as cookies.

And the vegetable oils used in the cookies or crackers may be more saturated than in their original form because they have been hydrogenated—treated under heat and pressure with hydrogen to keep them from turning rancid quickly, a process that converts unsaturated fats to saturated ones.

Getting enough of the right proteins

Unlike carbohydrates and fats, the third major class of food, proteins, are seldom needed to supply energy. Instead they are the chief building materials for skin, hair and nails; the structural components of muscles and ligaments; a major part of oxygen-carrying hemoglobin in the blood; and an essential constituent of internal organs such as the heart and brain. Proteins help form hormones, the chemical messengers of the body, enzymes, the compounds that facilitate digestion and other processes, and antibodies, the substances that combat foreign invaders threatening the body.

Proteins are a vital part of every cell. They are required in the greatest quantity when the body is building new tissue at a furious pace, as when a fetus is developing in the womb, or during infancy. Nursing mothers need extra protein; so do victims of burns, severe infection, blood loss or major surgery—all of which involve the loss of body protein. But the notion that athletic activity or strenuous exercise demands extra protein is a myth (exertion consumes energy, best supplied by carbohydrates or fats).

Similarly false is the idea that everyone must consume large amounts of protein-rich foods—meat, fish, fowl, eggs, cheese and so on—in order to build muscles and stay healthy. Most individuals need a relatively small proportion of their food in the form of proteins—about 10 per cent of all the calories in the diet should come from proteins. In most industrialized countries, the average intake is considerably higher—about 14 per cent of total calories. Just seven ounces of tuna, for example, will provide all the proteins an adult needs in a day. And two three-ounce hamburgers are more than enough for a child aged seven to 10.

There is an almost infinite number of compounds classified as proteins; all are constructed of very large molecules and all are made up of only 20 basic chemical building

The trick of living on vegetables alone

It is possible to live on nothing but vegetable foods, but it is not easy, and no large human society consumes a purely vegetarian diet. The reason is that vegetables are deficient in protein, which builds muscle, bone and skin. In a wholesome diet, about 10 per cent of the calories are proteins.

Not only do plants contain less protein than animal products; the proteins they do contain often are of a different kind. Vegetables generally lack some of the amino acids that the human body must have to make its own proteins. The body needs 20 amino acids. It can synthesize 12 of them, but it must get the other eight *(table)* directly from food. Only a very few vegetables, such as soybeans, supply all eight.

Thus anyone who wishes to survive on plant products alone must eat considerable amounts of vegetables that are rich in protein, and vegetables in combinations that supply the eight essential amino acids. The table shows how to meet both requirements. It lists vegetable foods that range from 3 to 40 per cent protein (for comparison, an egg is 12 per cent protein, tuna 28, roast beef 29); about ¾ cup of soybeans will satisfy both the protein and amino-acid requirements for a day and so will ½ cup each of pasta, split peas and sunflower seeds. But in addition, fats will be needed from nuts and seeds, and vitamins and minerals from leafy vegetables.

Achieving the proper balance without animal foods is tricky for adults, and small children may not be able to eat enough to avoid a dangerous protein deficiency.

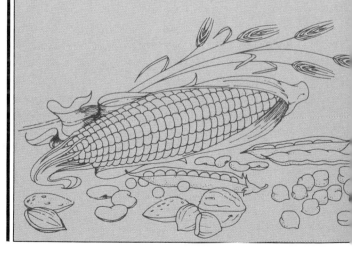

FOODS	Protein content	ESSENTIAL AMINO ACIDS							
		Isoleucine	Leucine	Lysine	Methionine	Phenylalanine	Threonine	Tryptophan	Valine
GRAINS									
Wheat germ	25%	●	●	●		●	●	●	●
Corn-soy grits	18%	●	●		●	●	●	●	●
Oatmeal	14%	●	●		●	●	●	●	●
Barley, pearl	13%	●	●		●	●		●	●
Bread, whole wheat	13%	●	●		●	●		●	●
Macaroni or spaghetti	13%	●	●		●	●		●	●
Wheat bran	12%	●	●		●	●		●	●
Millet	10%	●	●		●	●	●	●	●
Corn meal	9%	●	●		●	●	●		●
Rice	8%	●	●		●	●	●	●	●
Tortillas	6%	●	●				●		●
BEANS AND OTHER LEGUMES									
Soybeans	35%	●	●	●	●	●	●	●	●
Lupine	32%		●				●		●
Lentils	25%	●	●	●		●	●	●	●
Split peas	24%	●	●	●		●	●	●	●
Beans: navy, pea, pinto, red, or marrow	22%	●	●	●		●	●	●	●
Chickpeas	21%	●	●	●		●	●		●
Lima beans	21%	●	●	●		●	●	●	●
NUTS AND SEEDS									
Sesame meal	40%	●	●		●	●		●	
Peanuts	27%	●	●			●		●	●
Sunflower seeds	23%	●	●		●	●	●	●	●
Almonds	19%	●	●		●	●		●	●
Cashews	18%	●	●		●	●	●	●	●
Coconut	3%	●	●		●	●	●	●	●

The difficulty of meeting human needs for protein and amino acids from vegetables alone is indicated in this table, which lists typical foods in groups commonly used for planning a vegetarian diet. In each group, foods are listed in descending order of protein content; for each food, dots show the presence of essential amino acids in amounts considered adequate by the United Nations Food and Agriculture Organization. Fruits and green vegetables are omitted because most contain little protein.

blocks, called amino acids, that are assembled in a near-endless variety of combinations and permutations. Amino-acid molecules consist of atoms of nitrogen, hydrogen, carbon, oxygen, plus in some cases sulfur; it is these molecules that the body actually uses.

Supplying amino acids is the chief function of proteins. Digestion breaks down the proteins of food into their component amino acids, and other body processes then proceed to reassemble the amino acids into the myriad proteins humans need—huge molecules that may consist of thousands of the various amino acids woven together in chains, coils, spheres or basket shapes.

If food proteins do not supply all the amino acids the body requires, it can make some on its own. Internal chemical reactions convert certain amino acids into others and also synthesize some from the ingredients of fats and carbohydrates. However, eight amino acids that adults need cannot be manufactured in sufficient quantities by any process operating inside the human body. Consequently, these amino acids must be included, in large enough quantities, in the proteins that are eaten. And they must be furnished in the right proportions. If even one such essential amino acid is lacking in the diet for only a short time, its absence limits the production of proteins in the body.

Fortunately, many food proteins are considered complete, in the sense that they contain all eight of the essential amino acids and in about the right proportions. Such complete proteins are found mainly in animal foods—meats, eggs, milk and milk products. Most plant proteins are deficient in one or more of the essential amino acids, with the so-called limiting ingredient varying from plant to plant.

The average person does not need to count amino acids to ensure that he is getting adequate proteins. Even where meat and fish are scarce, all the essential amino acids are fairly easily acquired by combining small quantities of animal products—such as eggs or cheese—with certain plant products that contain considerable amounts of proteins. Proteins in animal products are not only complete but concentrated; thus a little suffices to make up for amino acids that may be insufficient in a diet derived mainly from plants. Getting by

on a little meat or fish, however, requires a choice of plant staples that meet two requirements. The plants must be rich in proteins. And they must be combined so that the amino acids missing from the proteins of one are supplied by the proteins of another.

This balancing act has long been performed by peoples all over the world. Since agriculture was invented about 10,000 years ago, the bulk of the human diet has consisted of grains—rice, wheat or millet bread, or corn tortillas, depending on which grass plant is available—served with legumes such as beans, peas or lentils. Any of these foods is a reasonably good source of proteins, but neither the grains nor the legumes suffice separately. The grains lack the essential amino acid lysine; legumes contain lysine but lack another essential amino acid called methionine—which grains have. Together grains and legumes make up nourishing dishes traditional in many cultures: tortillas and beans in Mexico, rice and beans *(arroz con gondules)* in Puerto Rico, rice and lentils *(kitcheri)* in India, rice and peas *(risi e bisi)* in Italy and the nuts and wheat that are eaten as peanut-butter sandwiches in modern America.

Although grains and legumes can supply all necessary proteins, to do so they must be eaten in large quantities. Even in whole-wheat bread, for example, protein supplies only 18 per cent of the energy; in tuna, it supplies 56 per cent. For this reason, most people who by choice or necessity live mainly on vegetables also eat some animal foods. The aborigines who live in Australia's Western Desert—"by any standard," wrote ethnographer R. A. Gould, it is one of the world's "most unreliable and impoverished" regions—are a remarkable example. They survive by gathering food. Women bring in 95 per cent of the diet; although mostly plants, it also includes small animals: lizards and mice.

The pure vegetable diet is rare—and dangerous unless very carefully planned and controlled for balance. One that was not balanced was the series of Zen macrobiotic diets adopted during the 1960s by some groups for a variety of reasons, including religious beliefs. To follow the program, the novice progressed through increasingly restricted levels of the diet, ending with little more than brown rice.

Diets such as these have caused serious illness and a few deaths. They are particularly dangerous to small children, who need larger quantities of the essential amino acids than do adults. It may be hard for small children to get enough protein from plant foods. Their original diet, mother's milk, is a rich protein source, and cow's milk or other high-protein food continues to be necessary during the early years of life. Children who do not get animal proteins—generally because their families cannot afford such foods—may suffer from retarded development, mental as well as physical.

In its extreme form, children's protein (and caloric) malnutrition, seen mainly in underdeveloped countries, is referred to as kwashiorkor. The origin of the word is instructive. In 1932 an English physician, Dr. Cecily Delphine Williams, wrote about a disease of young children that she thought might be caused by a shortage of certain amino acids. She found it in what is now called Ghana, and the word she used to describe it was the one used, with singular insight, by the Ga tribe. "Kwashiorkor" literally means "first-second." It overtakes the first-born child soon after weaning, which comes at the birth of a second child. The transition from mother's milk to a diet of starchy, low-protein vegetables, such as the cassava native to Africa, retards development, induces apathy and eventually may cause death. In some parts of India, Africa, Central and South America, and Southeast Asia, half the children die of kwashiorkor before their fifth birthday. Even in the United States the disease was seen in pockets of rural poverty in the South in the 1960s.

Fortunately, the course of kwashiorkor can be reversed, if caught early enough, by an improved diet. The mental retardation blamed on lesser protein deficiencies also seems to be reversible; if deprived children are put on a balanced diet and exposed to an intellectually stimulating environment, their mental aptitude approaches that of their well-fed peers.

What you need to know about vitamins

Except in areas of extreme poverty, people around the world get enough carbohydrates, fats and proteins. If they eat a variety of those macronutrients, they generally get sufficient micronutrients—vitamins and minerals—as well. The mi-

cronutrient balance, however, is more easily disturbed. Reliance on one foodstuff, particularly on such valuable sources of carbohydrates as corn or certain kinds of rice, may deprive the body of essential vitamins. Even geography has an effect—foods grown in certain parts of the world may lack needed minerals because the soil does not have enough.

Such deficiencies can bring on a variety of sometimes fatal illnesses, whose connection to diet was long elusive. Although the victims were obviously sick, it seemed that they were getting plenty to eat. Only when the cause of the illness was finally traced to food, in fact, was the existence of vitamins suspected.

Thirteen substances are now recognized as vitamins: dis-

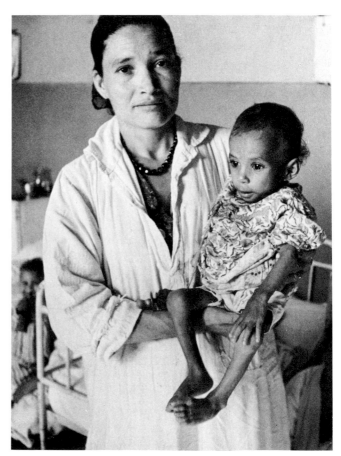

At Children's Hospital in Cairo, an anxious mother holds her son, his body withered by a form of malnutrition called marasmus. It is common in developing countries, where many babies are weaned before they can do without the rich proteins of mother's milk. The cure is simple and complete: protein-rich food.

tinct chemical compounds that must be present in food if it is to sustain health in human beings. They originally were identified by letter, and some still are, but all have been given names as more has been learned about their chemical compositions—vitamin C, for example, is now known to be the compound ascorbic acid.

Vitamins neither provide energy nor contribute any material to tissue building, but they are indispensable midwives to the creation of critical components of the body, from blood cells to genes. They act as catalysts to assist the chemicals called enzymes in the transformation of the macronutrients into energy and body tissues. Vitamins and enzymes help a chemical process get started and control its speed, but are not used up. All the vitamins that are needed in a day amount to a mere fiftieth of a teaspoon. Just one ounce of one kind of B vitamin would fill the daily needs of 9,450,000 people. The amounts of vitamins required every day are so small they are generally specified in milligrams (.000035 ounce) or micrograms (.000000035 ounce).

Four vitamins—A, D, E and K—are soluble in fat and insoluble in water. They usually enter the body with fatty foods and vegetables, are stored in body fat and in the liver in modest quantities when not needed, and therefore do not have to be included in each day's meals. The other nine vitamins—vitamin C plus eight of the B vitamin family—dissolve in water and are not stored in the body in substantial amounts. Any surplus is excreted in the urine. (Some experts wryly note that those who consume massive doses of these vitamins have the most expensive urine in the world.) Because they are not stored, these vitamins should be included, in adequate amounts, in each day's diet.

The biochemical roles of these 13 vitamins have now been identified, and the vitamins isolated and synthesized in pure form. But this is a fairly recent development, the culmination of centuries of frustrating speculation and trials.

By the end of the 17th Century many ship's surgeons recognized that the lack of fresh fruits and vegetables on long voyages led to the debilitating, often fatal disease of scurvy, and by 1753 the British physician James Lind proved with a controlled experiment that people could avoid scurvy by drinking citrus juices. But it was not until 1928 that the crucial scurvy preventive so plentiful in citrus fruits, vitamin C, was isolated and identified as ascorbic acid.

Similarly, the disease called pellagra ("rough skin" in Italian, after a typical symptom of this debilitating ailment) broke out in Europe after explorers returning from the New World introduced corn as a major crop; as early as 1795 pellagra was linked to a corn diet by the Italian physician Giuseppi Cerri. He noticed that pellagra struck mainly rural villagers, who subsisted largely on cornmeal. He put 10 victims on the more varied diet of city folk, and they got well; when they went back to the usual village diet of cornmeal, they came down with pellagra again. Not until the early 20th Century, after Dr. Joseph Goldberger of the United States Public Health Service conducted extensive studies in the pellagra-plagued South and experimented on human volunteers in a Mississippi prison, was there proof of the connection between the ailment and the lack of an essential ingredient in corn. And not until 1937 was the ingredient identified as niacin, one of the B vitamin family.

The difficulty of uncovering the truth about vitamins is perhaps best illustrated by the story of the B vitamin thiamine, a lack of which produces the disease called beriberi. Beriberi attacks the nervous system and the heart, and can result in paralysis and death. Discovery of its link with thiamine was the culmination of a series of experiments in places as disparate as a Javanese chicken yard, Japanese Navy vessels and European research hospitals.

Beriberi had ravaged the Far East for millennia—it was reported in China in 2600 B.C.—when in the late 19th Century newly developed techniques of medical science were applied to finding its cause and cure. One hero of the story is a young physician in the Japanese Navy, Dr. K. Takaki, trained in London and appointed director of the Tokyo Naval Hospital (and eventually made a baron). Dr. Takaki was appalled when a training ship named the *Rinjio* returned in 1884 from an around-the-world cruise with 169 of its crew suffering from beriberi; 25 died. He thereupon talked the Admiralty into experiments "upon a scale of great magnitude." He had deduced that the lack of some essential food-

A daily budget of vitamins and minerals

The details of daily requirements of vitamins and minerals, as listed for adult males in the table below and overleaf, indicate why there is so much confusion about the proper amounts required by humans. Most nutrition authorities maintain that the average person gets more than enough of the essential nutrients simply by eating a variety of common foods. Yet the amounts given may seem to be more than many people ordinarily consume. In fact, very few people in the industrialized world suffer for lack of vitamins or minerals.

The minimums leave a large margin for error. Most vitamins and minerals occur in many foods. Some vitamins are made in the body and need not be supplied by food. Certain foods—cereals, milk and butter—are artificially enriched with many ingredients.

However, these protections can fail. Children and pregnant women need more of certain ingredients than most adults. Vegetarians risk vitamin B_{12} deficiency and people who shun fruits and green vegetables may not receive enough vitamin C. Medical treatments can block the absorption of certain vitamins and minerals. Illness upsets the body's own vitamin-making processes. Nearly all such deficiencies are best remedied by altering the diet.

VITAMIN	Richest food sources	Important body functions	Suggested daily amount	
ASCORBIC ACID: VITAMIN C	Citrus fruits and juices, strawberries, cantaloupes, tomatoes, peppers, leafy vegetables, potatoes	Promotes growth of skin, bones, tendons and supportive tissue	60 mg., equivalent to 1 serving of grapefruit juice	When taken with iron, vitamin C permits more of the iron to be absorbed and used by the body.
VITAMIN B_{12}	All animal products, but highly concentrated in liver	Essential to the functioning of all cells	.003 mg., equivalent to 1 large serving of ground beef and 1 cup of milk	Because no vitamin B_{12} is present in plant products, vegetarians risk deficiency.
BIOTIN	Meats, vegetables, milk, mushrooms, peanuts, bananas, grapefruit	Helps convert fats and carbohydrates into protein and energy for the body	.1 to .2 mg., equivalent to 2 servings of meat and 4 servings of fruit or vegetables	
VITAMIN D	Fish liver oils, milk, eggs, tuna, sardines	Helps body absorb calcium and phosphorus to promote growth of strong bones	.005 mg., equivalent to 2 cups of milk	The adult need can be met by normal exposure to sunlight. Children, as well as pregnant women and nursing mothers, need twice the normal adult amount of vitamin D.
FOLACIN	Legumes, liver, leafy vegetables, eggs, asparagus, bananas, orange juice	Prevents blood disorders; helps body use proteins	.4 mg., equivalent to 1 serving of chicken liver	Even with a normal diet, folacin deficiency is common among pregnant women, who need twice the normal adult amount.
VITAMIN K	Leafy vegetables, fruits, eggs, cauliflower, cereals	Maintains normal blood clotting	.07 to .14 mg., equivalent to 4 servings of fruit or vegetables	The body manufactures its own vitamin K, so that even those who shun fruits and vegetables are rarely deficient.
NIACIN	Liver, lean meats, fish, poultry, breads and cereals, vegetables, peanuts	Helps convert food into energy	18 mg., equivalent to 2 servings of meat or poultry	Large amounts—sometimes prescribed for people suffering from blood-vessel disease—may produce a burning sensation or a red rash around the neck, face and hands.
PANTOTHENIC ACID	Liver, eggs, potatoes, broccoli, dairy products, fruits	Helps convert food into energy	4 to 7 mg., equivalent to 2 scrambled eggs and 1 serving of broccoli	

Only the richest sources of vitamins and minerals are listed in the table above and overleaf; many other foods are good sources. The suggested amounts are generous for most adults; children and pregnant or nursing mothers generally require more.

VITAMIN	Richest food sources	Important body functions	Suggested daily amount	
PYRIDOXINE: VITAMIN B_6	Chicken, fish, vegetables, whole-grain cereals, potatoes, bananas	Regenerates red blood cells; maintains normal functioning of nervous tissues	2.2 mg., equivalent to 1 serving of chicken, 2 servings of vegetables and 1 banana	
RETINOL: VITAMIN A	Liver, carrots, spinach, collards, sweet potatoes, milk, cheese, eggs, apricots, cantaloupes, peaches	Prevents night blindness; maintains mucous membranes and skin; promotes normal growth of bones and teeth	1 mg., equivalent to 1 serving of spinach and 1 serving of diced carrots	Consuming more than 7.5 mg. daily for long periods of time may cause headaches, vomiting or loss of hair.
RIBOFLAVIN: VITAMIN B_2	Meats, fish, poultry, milk, cheese, eggs, leafy vegetables, breads and cereals	Promotes healthy skin, eyes and nerves; aids reactions that provide energy	1.6 mg., equivalent to 1 serving of beef liver	
THIAMINE: VITAMIN B_1	Pork, organ meats, fish, poultry, breads and cereals, eggs, leafy vegetables, legumes, nuts	Aids reactions that provide energy to the body; promotes normal appetite and digestion; aids in transmission of nerve impulses	1.4 mg., equivalent to 1 serving of pork or 1 serving of peas	Tea contains a chemical that opposes the beneficial action of thiamine.
TOCOPHEROL: VITAMIN E	Vegetable oils, liver, eggs, margarine	Helps the body utilize other compounds such as vitamin A; essential to proper functioning of blood	10 mg., equivalent to 2 tablespoons mayonnaise or vegetable oil	

MINERAL	Richest food sources	Important body functions	Suggested daily amount	
CALCIUM	Milk, cheese, turnip greens, broccoli, kale, citrus fruits, sardines	Essential for blood clotting, heart and muscle function, development of healthy bones and teeth	800 mg., equivalent to 2 cups of milk, ½ cup of leafy vegetable and 1 orange	For the efficient absorption of calcium in the body, adequate consumption of vitamin D is necessary.
CHLORINE	Table salt (sodium chloride), almost all foods	Helps the blood carry carbon dioxide to the lungs; an essential component of digestive fluids	1,700 to 5,100 mg. (ordinary foods contain so much salt that nearly everyone gets an excess of chlorine)	Because sodium in salt influences heart, kidney and liver diseases, persons with such ailments may have to reduce salt consumption and make up for the loss of chlorine by taking other compounds containing it.
CHROMIUM	Meats, vegetable oils, whole-grain breads and cereals, cheese, beer	Stimulates enzymes that produce energy; helps regulate insulin levels	.05 to .2 mg., equivalent to 1 serving of puffed-rice cereal	
COPPER	Oysters, nuts, liver, mushrooms, gelatin, whole-grain breads and cereals	Helps produce hemoglobin, which carries oxygen in the blood	2 to 3 mg., equivalent to 1 serving of raw mushrooms and 1 serving of corn	Premature infants are born with low copper reserves, and special formulas are needed to overcome the deficiency.
FLUORINE	Fluoridated drinking water, tea, fish	Helps form healthy bones and tooth enamel	1.5 to 4 mg., equivalent to 3 cups of tea	About half the U.S. water supply is fluoridated; people who drink water containing about 1 part fluorine per million have 50 per cent less tooth decay than those drinking unfluoridated water.

MINERAL	Richest food sources	Important body functions	Suggested daily amount	
IODINE	Fish, iodized table salt	Maintains proper functioning of the thyroid gland; lack of iodine causes goiter	.15 mg. (ordinary foods contain so much iodized salt that nearly everyone gets an excess of iodine)	Those on salt-free diets generally obtain sufficient iodine from milk and meats from animals given iodized feed.
IRON	Liver, meats, poultry, fish, leafy vegetables, beans	Essential component of hemoglobin, which carries oxygen in the blood; lack of iron causes anemia	10 mg., equivalent to 1 serving of liver, or 1 serving of chicken plus 1 serving of leafy vegetable	As many as one out of four Americans may suffer from iron deficiency. Women of child-bearing age need twice as much iron as men because of blood loss during menstruation. During pregnancy, as much as 60 mg. per day may be needed, and supplements are commonly prescribed for pregnant women.
MAGNESIUM	Milk, cheese, poultry, whole-grain breads and cereals, vegetables	Activates enzymes that supply energy to the body; regulates body temperature	350 mg., equivalent to 4 servings of vegetables	
MANGANESE	Tea, whole-grain breads and cereals, vegetables, fruits, nuts	Helps convert carbohydrates and fats into protein and energy for the body; aids in development of the pancreas	2.5 to 5 mg., equivalent to 3 cups of tea	
MOLYBDENUM	Organ meats, legumes, cereals	Helps convert waste chemicals into urine	.15 to .5 mg., equivalent to 1 serving of green beans	Daily intake of 10 to 15 mg. over a long period may cause a goutlike illness; molybdenum supplements are not recommended.
PHOSPHORUS	Meats, cheese, poultry, fish, whole-grain breads and cereals, eggs, nuts, legumes	Combines with calcium to form bones and teeth; helps regulate many body functions	800 mg., equivalent to 1 glass of milk, 1 serving of sole, 1 serving of beef and 1 serving of cheddar cheese	Antacid stomach remedies may hinder the absorption of phosphorus.
POTASSIUM	Orange juice, milk, meats, vegetables, bananas, prunes, raisins	Balances fluid levels within cells	1,875 to 5,625 mg., equivalent to 1 glass of orange juice	Diarrhea, or the use of certain diuretics, blood-pressure pills, or laxatives, may cause a deficiency. A sudden excessive intake of potassium—about 18,000 mg.—can cause a heart attack.
SELENIUM	Fish, meats, breads and cereals	Necessary to proper functioning of blood	.05 to .2 mg., equivalent to 1 serving of salmon	Excess selenium from mineral supplements may cause skin rashes, loss of hair and tooth decay.
SODIUM	Table salt (sodium chloride), almost all foods	Regulates amounts of water and other fluids in the body and thus influences blood pressure; essential to nerve impulse transmission, and to energy production	1,100 to 3,300 mg. (ordinary foods contain so much salt that nearly everyone gets an excess of sodium)	Much sodium is consumed from nonfood sources, such as antacid stomach remedies. Excess sodium is blamed for arterial diseases.
ZINC	Meats, fish, eggs	Promotes growth of tissues; prevents anemia; helps heal wounds	15 mg., equivalent to 1 serving of oysters	Vegetarians risk zinc deficiency.

stuff had caused beriberi aboard the *Rinjio*. To test this idea, he later wrote, "the *Taukuba*, a training ship, was then sent out to follow the same course as that the *Rinjio* had taken," so that influences of climate would be the same. But the *Taukuba* departed with stores of meats and vegetables as well as the rice that had sustained the *Rinjio's* men.

"There was not a death from disease during the whole voyage," reported Dr. Takaki. Meals throughout the Navy were immediately upgraded, and the incidence of beriberi—1,979 cases in 1879—dropped to zero by 1887.

Although Dr. Takaki correctly recognized that beriberi was caused by a dietary deficiency, he incorrectly assumed the problem was one of too few proteins. The proteins added to the Japanese sailors' diet simply made up for the deficiency in their staple, rice. Polished rice was singled out as the culprit by a team of Dutch physicians, unacquainted with Dr. Takaki's research, who were sent to the Dutch colony of Java to attack the beriberi problem there.

They assumed they were looking for bacteria as a cause of beriberi, and one young member of the group, Dr. Christiaan Eijkman, experimented on chickens. To economize, he fed them scraps from the food served in a military hospital. He quickly noticed that the chickens began to stagger around the yard, obviously suffering from a nervous-system ailment akin to that symptomatic of beriberi. Then a new director took charge of the hospital, and he refused to provide table scraps for the chickens. Dr. Eijkman substituted unmilled rice as chicken feed—and the animals promptly recovered. In 1896, he and another member of the group compared milled and unmilled rice in experiments on humans. Prisoners fed polished rice, or rice with its outer coats removed by milling, came down with beriberi. Those who were given unmilled rice did not.

The Dutch team realized that something in the outer coats of rice prevented beriberi. Dr. Eijkman thought it was a substance that counteracted a poison present in the rice kernel. After years of study, Dr. Gerrit Grijns suggested the true answer: The outer coats of rice contain an essential nutrient.

In 1912, Casimir Funk, a Polish-born chemist, extracted from the outer coats a substance that seemed to be the vital ingredient. It was a type of compound called an amine—a nitrogen-containing compound. Funk suggested that there was a whole class of such vital amines, which he named vitamines, which in small amounts prevent beriberi and other deficiency diseases such as scurvy and pellagra. The beriberi preventive is indeed an amine, thiamine, finally isolated in pure form in 1926. Funk was wrong about the other vitamins, however; many are not amines but a variety of chemical types, and to avoid confusion, the "e" was eventually dropped from the name.

Elusive minerals

The search for the vitamins was intense because the ailments caused by a lack of them are serious and obvious. Generally more subtle are the results of deficiencies in the other minute ingredients necessary in healthful food, the minerals. Some are needed in relatively large amounts, as much as .2 ounce per day. These "major minerals" include calcium, phosphorus, sodium, chlorine, potassium, magnesium and sulfur. Others, the "trace minerals," are needed in far smaller amounts. They include manganese, iron, copper, iodine, zinc, fluorine, and perhaps many others—the number of essential minerals is past 20 and growing.

The role of minerals in the body is extremely varied, and that of the trace minerals is not completely understood. Calcium and phosphorus are essential for the building of healthy bones and teeth. (There are more than 2½ pounds of calcium in the body of a 160-pound man, 98 per cent of it contained in his bones.) But calcium also helps to regulate blood clotting and muscle action.

Among the trace minerals, fluorine clearly helps prevent tooth decay, but the part manganese plays is not established. Iodine is essential for the normal functioning of the thyroid gland. When not enough iodine is present in the diet, the gland enlarges into what is called a goiter, an unsightly swelling of the neck that can interfere with speech and breathing. Goiter was once prevalent in the midwestern United States, but today is most common among isolated mountain people. Ranges like the Himalayas and the Andes have little access to foods from the sea, the richest source of iodine.

Goiter was essentially eliminated from the United States in the same way that many other deficiency diseases were eradicated from much of the world: by adding essential vitamins and minerals to common foodstuffs. Most of the salt sold in industrialized countries contains added iodine so that when it is used for seasoning it prevents goiter. White bread contains added niacin, thiamine, riboflavin and iron so that normal consumption of bread prevents pellagra and beriberi. Milk contains added vitamin D, needed by children to prevent the bone-deforming disease, rickets. Margarine contains added vitamin A, which aids vision at night, is essential for growth and maintains healthy tissue.

And yet, not everyone who eats what is considered a balanced diet gets enough of all the essential vitamins and minerals; among those with special needs are pregnant women, nursing mothers, infants, the elderly, women taking oral contraceptives, and people on low-calorie reducing diets. Of particular concern to these groups are two vitamins and three minerals: folacin, vitamin B_6, iron, magnesium and zinc. These can be obtained in sufficient quantities from an ordinary day's meals, however, if certain foods are included:

- For folacin: legumes, liver, leafy vegetables, eggs, asparagus, bananas, or orange juice.
- For vitamin B_6: chicken, fish, liver, vegetables, whole-grain cereals, potatoes, or bananas.
- For iron: liver, meat, poultry, fish, leafy vegetables, lima beans, dried apricots, or raisins.
- For magnesium: milk, cheese, poultry, pecans, or whole-grain breads and cereals.
- For zinc: meat, fish, or eggs.

The most common deficiency among ordinarily well-fed people is in the mineral iron, which among other functions forms part of the hemoglobin that carries oxygen in the blood; a lack of iron brings on the lassitude of anemia. A survey in 1977 and 1978 found that the average iron intake among American women of child-bearing age was 35 to 40 per cent less than the amount recommended. Their iron deficiency was presumably caused by loss of blood during menstruation. But extra iron is also required during pregnancy, when development of the fetus and placenta calls for the transfer of large stores of iron from the mother's body. And the elderly, because they eat less, may also lack iron. In a study conducted by the U.S. Department of Health, Education and Welfare, 40 per cent of the men and 66 per cent of the women among those 65 years of age and older were found to be getting less iron than the recommended standard.

Less widely recognized is the need for extra minerals and vitamins induced by certain medical treatments. Such marginal deficiencies may be "a surprisingly common problem," according to Dr. Richard Rivlin, Chief of the Nutrition Division of New York Hospital-Cornell Medical Center in New York City. Prolonged treatment with certain drugs, as well as some hormone disorders, can interfere with the body's utilization of what would otherwise be an adequate amount of vitamins from food.

For example, the antidepressant drug chlorpromazine, which is taken over long periods of time by large numbers of patients with emotional disorders, interferes with the use of

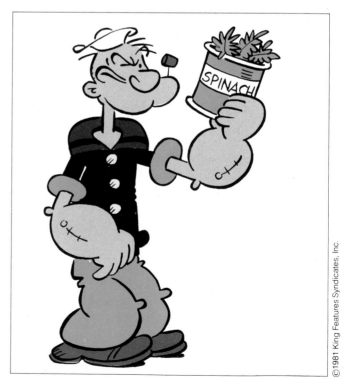

©1981 King Features Syndicates, Inc.

Popeye the Sailor, the feisty cartoon hero, endeared himself to nutrition-conscious parents by inspiring youngsters to eat mineral-rich spinach. But Popeye's efforts may have been misguided. Kenneth Lee of the University of Wisconsin found that although spinach does contain iron, it also contains a chemical that prevents the body from absorbing very much.

the vitamin riboflavin. The drug boric acid—present in some 400 products commonly used in the home, including mouthwashes—also interferes with riboflavin; Dr. Rivlin believes that even small amounts of boric acid ingested over a long time can result in a marginal deficiency of the vitamin.

Oral contraceptives may decrease the need for iron but increase the need for B vitamins. Even laxatives can interfere with vitamin absorption if used for prolonged periods.

Beyond these medical side effects, deficiencies of vitamins and minerals may occur simply because not everyone eats a well-balanced, nutritious diet. Many teenagers adopt rather bizarre eating habits, and many grownups in a high-pressure society eat erratically. Dieters, whose daily intake may drop below 1,200 calories, may not get enough vitamins and minerals because the quantity and often the variety of their food are limited. The elderly, who generally eat less because of decreased activity, are also susceptible to vitamin deficiencies. Infants, small children, pregnant women and nursing mothers may also have unusually high requirements that are not met by an otherwise nutritious diet.

Dangers in supplements

For any of these reasons, supplements—vitamin or mineral pills, protein concentrates, or extra fiber—may be needed. If they are not needed—and most authorities think they generally are not—the moderate amounts added by the typical vitamin-mineral pills are, for most people, relatively harmless insurance against deficiencies *(pages 43-45)*. Some individuals, however, consume huge quantities of vitamins and other food supplements, amounts that far exceed the allotments considered advisable for good health. An excess can be a greater health hazard than a deficiency.

People go on vitamin binges partly as a result of new scientific findings—tentative, preliminary data that serve as a jumping-off point for unlikely conclusions. Vitamin E, for example, was shown to prevent the destruction of certain tissues. Tissue deterioration is one aspect of aging. Some people put those two facts together to reach the conclusion, unsupported by any real evidence, that vitamin E slows the aging process. One prominent proponent of vitamin E

(whose Ph.D. degree came from a Nevada diploma mill) urged daily doses 40 times greater than those believed necessary for healthy tissue. The fact is that a surplus of vitamin E may have serious ill effects: It may slow the clotting of blood, apparently by interfering with the utilization of vitamin K.

Most vitamins pose some danger if taken in very large quantities. Both vitamin A and vitamin D can be poisonous in large doses. Too much vitamin A causes a variety of afflictions, from headache to swelling of the legs; too much vitamin D brings on vomiting, diarrhea and kidney damage. The effects can be cumulative, because both these vitamins, soluble in fat, are stored in the liver. Indeed, polar-bear livers contain so much vitamin A that they have poisoned Arctic explorers who subsisted on them.

It would be almost impossible to get sick on the vitamins in an ordinary diet, though common foods are artificially enriched with them. But it is possible to get too much by over-enthusiastic consumption of vitamin pills or of certain foods.

One overprotective Michigan mother almost killed her three-year-old daughter by giving her huge doses of vitamin A—100 times the amount recommended—in a misguided attempt to ward off winter colds. The child was hospitalized with kidney and liver damage, and narrowly survived.

Even water-soluble vitamins, which are not stored in the body, can be hazardous when taken in excess. Some authorities are concerned that large doses of vitamin C, taken in the belief they prevent colds, can affect bone development, and the ability of the white blood cells to kill bacteria. Large doses have caused severe diarrhea in some individuals, and are suspected as causes of kidney stones.

Even when the results of an overdose of vitamins are not unhealthful, they can be embarrassing. Witness the strange case of the orange man. The man startled, then baffled his physician because his skin was a bright, glowing orange—an unheard-of color. The puzzle was finally solved when the patient revealed that, through a desire for maximum vitamin intake, he had developed a passion for their natural source, vegetables. He ate carrots all day long, and tomato juice was his favorite drink. Together, these vegetables supplied him not only with more than enough vitamins A and C, but also with much yellow pigment (carotene from carrots) and red pigment (lycopene from tomatoes). The orange man went down in the medical books as the first recorded case of carotenemia-lycopenemia.

But not the last. A woman with the same orange skin turned up in the same doctor's office four years later. She ate substantial amounts of carrots and tomatoes every day.

Mineral supplements can also be overindulged in. Large amounts of zinc can cause heart disease by interfering with the body's use of copper, according to Dr. Walter Mertz of the U.S. Department of Agriculture: "At a certain level, not overly high, zinc can interact with other essential trace elements, notably copper. You can produce a relative copper deficiency. Unfortunately, at present, it just happens to not be fashionable to swallow copper also."

The attempt to obtain large amounts of calcium from supplements has resulted in serious illness in numbers of cases—though not from the calcium. Some health enthusiasts downed quantities of dolomite, a natural, white mineral that contains both calcium and magnesium. They became sick because dolomite can also contain such very toxic metals as lead, arsenic and mercury, which derange the nervous system, causing confusion, nausea, vomiting and diarrhea.

Even the effort to eradicate goiter in inland America by adding iodine to table salt has backfired in some cases. Too much can cause goiter as well as too little. Surveys of foods eaten in 1974 and 1975 discovered that many Americans were getting about five times more iodine than they needed, and babies were receiving as much as 13 times more. Most of the excess came from milk—cattle feed and salt licks contained added iodine, and milk absorbed some iodine from a disinfectant widely used in dairies. But foods flavored with salt and other iodized seasonings also played a role. A typical fast-food meal—hamburger, fried potatoes and milk shake —provides three times the daily allotment of iodine.

The essential nutrients: How much is just right?

One reason some people suffer from a lack of essential nutrients—proteins, carbohydrates and fats as well as vitamins or minerals—while others suffer from an excess is the uncertainty over what the proper daily allotments should be. There is a consensus on how much of what is too little and how much is too much, but there is little agreement about how much is just right.

Many countries have their own recommendations for a satisfactory allotment of nutrients, and they vary widely, influenced partly by economics (wealthy nations set the standards high), but mainly by scientific disagreement.

In the 1960s, for example, the Canadian allotment of proteins for young men was about 15 per cent lower than the allotment of the United States, and about 19 per cent lower than the standards set by the United Kingdom, as well as by the United Nations.

On the other hand, the United States calcium allowance was about 50 per cent higher than the allowances set by the United Nations, Canada and Britain, although all of them were apparently based on the same experimental data. Explained D. Mark Hegsted, Administrator for Human Nutrition of the U.S. Department of Agriculture: "A country with a restricted food supply can't be as liberal as others. It needs stronger evidence of a genuine need for high levels. Calcium is one example. America has a very large milk supply. But if milk supplies were limited, setting the calcium allowances high would create many problems."

Such divergences of authoritative opinion stem from the difficulty of establishing required amounts. Animal tests are of limited help because the food needs of each species are unique—rats and rabbits, for example, do not require vitamin C from food; they make it in their bodies. Tests on humans to identify minimum limits were used in the past but are no longer permitted because they could harm the subjects. One way out of this dilemma relies on averages. The diets of average, healthy people are analyzed, and the ingredients those people take in are assumed to be about right for other people like them.

A more elaborate evaluation of food needs is provided by the so-called balance study, used in measuring requirements for minerals *(pages 52-63)*. The study is based on the fact that the amount of each chemical element present inside the body of a healthy adult remains essentially the same so long as he

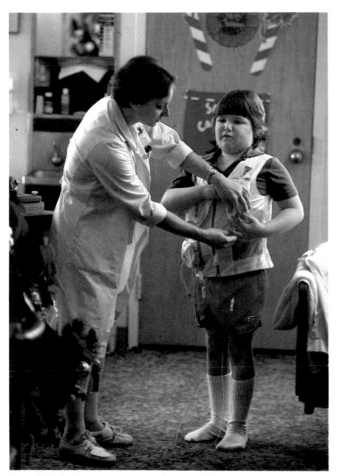

At a clinic in Houston a nurse adjusts a lifesaving garment called a total parenteral nutrition vest for a 10-year-old boy who has an ulcer so severe that he cannot take food or drink by mouth. The vest, in effect, feeds him: Nutrient fluids stored in plastic pouches are forced through tubes and a needle by a battery-powered pump, and enter his bloodstream near his heart.

does not lose or gain weight. The calcium he consumes in his food, for example, will be made by metabolic processes into various compounds needed for bodily repair and operation; after those compounds serve their purposes, the calcium passes into wastes that are excreted. In the case of calcium, the waste might include worn-out bone substances that have been replaced by the fresh calcium just consumed. Some of the fresh calcium may be kept inside the body as a reserve that can be drawn upon when insufficient calcium is consumed. But the size of the reserve is more or less fixed. Thus a healthy adult excretes as much calcium as he consumes— provided he consumes neither more nor less than his body needs to operate normally.

In balance experiments, volunteers are fed carefully measured meals that contain slightly more or less of a single essential ingredient; then the amount of that ingredient excreted—in urine, feces and sweat—is measured. If the volunteer excretes as much of the substance as he eats, his body is getting just enough. If he excretes more than he eats, he is drawing on body reserves to maintain metabolic operation— and he is eating less than he needs. If he excretes less than he eats, he must be storing some in his body and he is getting more than just enough of the ingredient in his food.

Such methods obviously allow for great latitude in interpretation of the results. In the United States the data are reviewed every five years by the Food and Nutrition Board of the National Research Council, an independent but semi-official agency. The Board issues Recommended Dietary Allowances for many food ingredients considered essential. This RDA list changes over time; it included 10 substances in 1943, 17 in 1968 and 18 by 1980. For many other ingredients that still have been only partially evaluated—including several minerals—the Board has issued estimates of ''safe and adequate'' amounts.

Because carbohydrates and fats are both primarily energy sources, the 1980 list did not specify separate quantities for these macronutrients, but simply gave an energy allowance in calories; it did not make a specific recommendation for the ratio of carbohydrates to fats. The RDA list did specify quantities for protein, for 10 vitamins, and for six minerals. These amounts were broken down into 15 categories by sex and age, and separate amounts were established for pregnant or lactating women.

Such standards, established to aid in maintaining health among large population groups, obviously cannot take into account variations in the needs of individuals. In any case the RDAs, as issued by the semiofficial National Research Council, are too cumbersome for general use. They are not the ones that are indicated on food packages. Those are USRDAs, promulgated by an official part of the federal government, the Food and Drug Administration. The USRDAs are based on the RDAs, but they are not broken down by age and sex. They list only one value, generally the highest of all, for any nutrient given by the RDA. So the package labels are likely to overstate considerably the amounts needed by most individuals. Many foodstuffs, of course, are not packaged, and their nutrient contents must be ascertained from tables—the important ingredients in 290 foods are listed on pages 160-171, and a table on pages 43-45 details specific requirements for 28 vitamins and minerals.

Such data can serve as a guide in planning meals that will meet individual needs. An assortment of foods should be selected so that each day's meals will include several items from a few basic groups:

● Vegetables and fruits. Eat four servings—about ½ cup each—every day. (In these allowances servings generally, but not always, correspond to the portions of food listed in the chart on pages 160-171.) Choose dark green vegetables (spinach, green peppers, kale, broccoli, parsley, watercress), tomatoes, and citrus fruits or juice for vitamin C. Yellow or orange vegetables (sweet potatoes, carrots, winter squash) and leafy greens (chard, spinach, kale) provide vitamin A. For fiber, rely on unpeeled fruits and vegetables, and those with edible seeds, such as berries.

● Breads and cereals. Eat four servings daily. One serving consists of one slice of bread; ½ to ¾ cup of cooked cereal, cornmeal or pasta; or one cup of ready-to-eat cereal. At least some of these foods should be whole-grain products, which contribute fiber, vitamins and minerals that are lost when whole grains are milled in the refining process.

● Milk and cheese. The number of servings recommended depends partly on age: Children under nine need two or three servings, children aged nine to 12 three servings, teenagers four servings, and adults two servings. However, pregnant women should eat three servings and nursing mothers four servings. One serving is an eight-ounce glass of milk, one cup of yogurt or 1⅓ ounces of cheese. Such milk products are a major source of calcium, protein and vitamin D, and also provide other vitamins. Fortified skim milk and low-fat milk have essentially the same nutrients as whole milk, but of course less fat and fewer calories.

● Meat, poultry, fish and beans. Eat two servings daily. A serving consists of two to three ounces of meat, poultry or fish, two eggs, one to two cups of cooked beans, four tablespoons of peanut butter, or about ½ to one cup of nuts or seeds. Foods in this group are valuable sources of protein, vitamins and minerals. But there is wide variation in their ingredients and an assortment is required. It would be a poor idea, for example, to eat nothing but red meat from among these foods. Red meats are good sources of zinc. But liver and egg yolks are high in vitamin A; nuts are rich in magnesium; and seeds contribute essential fatty acids. Vitamin B_{12} occurs only in foods of animal origin (although some vegetable products produced expressly for pure vegetarians are artificially fortified with this vitamin).

The number of servings suggested for adults from these four food groups will supply adequate amounts of proteins and many vitamins and minerals, but only about 1,200 calories a day. That many calories may suffice for some sedentary adults, or for individuals on reducing diets, but not for most active people. To include enough calories, increase the portion size and eat some of the fats and sweets that add flavor to meals—candy, sugar, jellies, soft drinks, butter, pastry and salad dressings. But eat no more than enough to keep weight at the desired level.

When meals are made up in this way—selected from a variety of vegetables, meats and grains plus dollops of tasty fats and sweets—pills and special supplements are seldom needed. Traditional dishes provide all the nutrients the average person needs—and enjoyable eating as well. ❋

Chris Gruver, a volunteer test subject at the Human Nutrition Laboratory, laps up a spill on his lunch tray to get every last bit of his calibrated diet. A competitive cyclist in "civilian" life and thus accustomed to a hefty intake of some 5,500 calories a day, he exercises and eats as much as he usually would, although for the purposes of testing, the composition of his meals varies.

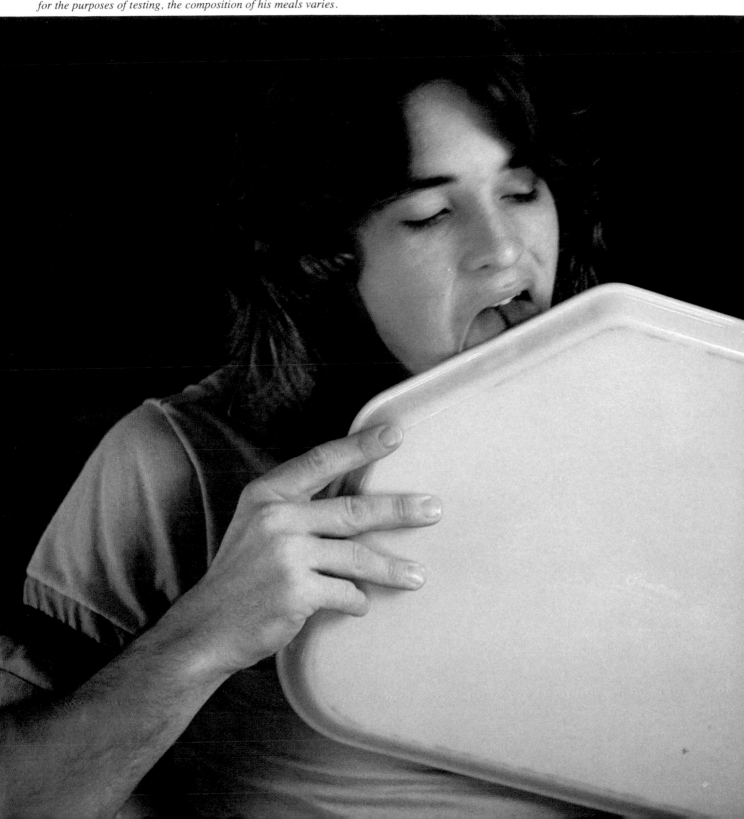

Prospecting for trace minerals in daily fare

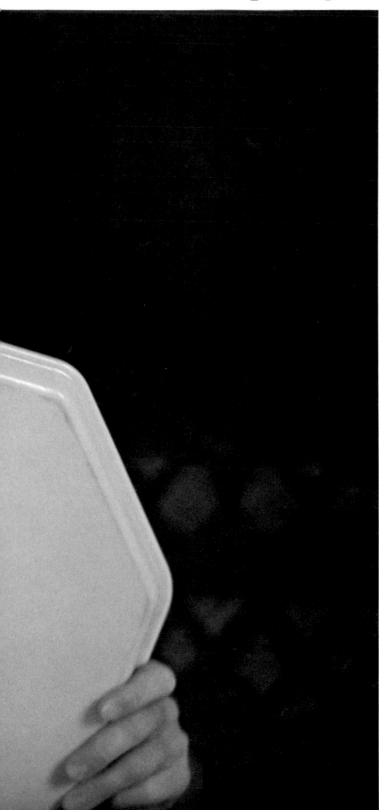

Some minerals the body needs to stay healthy are required in such small amounts that only elaborate research can figure out how much is too much or too little. Just .00007 ounce of copper, for example, should be present in a day's meals. A great deal less brings on anemia; more causes nausea and vomiting.

There may be as many as 15 essential dietary trace elements. The amounts needed seem to vary with the balance of particular kinds of fats, proteins and carbohydrates. The only way to track trace elements accurately is to study humans the way scientists study rats—in a laboratory. Remarkably, a laboratory that studies humans actually exists, in Grand Forks, North Dakota, and the "human rats" who live and work there do so voluntarily.

Called the Human Nutrition Laboratory, it was established in 1970 by the U.S. Department of Agriculture at the University of North Dakota. Its staff of physicians, biochemists, microbiologists, nutritionists, dieticians, nurses and psychologists monitor as many as eight live-in male recruits at a time, all of them surviving on experimental diets.

Each volunteer is screened for his ability to withstand tests, and those selected are paid a nominal fee. In exchange, each must live a monklike existence for three to six months, leave the building only in the company of a chaperon, and be on call virtually 24 hours a day. He must eat and drink exactly what is prescribed, no more, no less—sometimes literally licking the platter clean *(left)*.

All meals are prepared in the center's own kitchen from foods of known composition: bread from a USDA laboratory, distilled water, beef from identical steers in the university herd, vegetables frozen or canned in the same lot. Everything is weighed, then cooked in two containers, one portion to be eaten, the duplicate to be set aside for analysis *(see pages 62-63)*. Alcoholic drinks, cigarettes, candy and many toothpastes are forbidden; so are shampoos and hand soaps that might be absorbed by the body. The seemingly innocent act of licking a stamp is outlawed—mucilage might add unprogramed chemicals to the system.

So that researchers can gauge the consumption of trace minerals, subjects must collect body wastes. Even hair clippings and sweat are saved. Blood tests, checks on weight *(pages 54-55)*, heart and brain-wave recordings *(pages 58-59)* and psychological tests help reveal changes in body functions caused by variations in trace minerals in the diets.

Among discoveries emerging from this research is the importance of zinc, found essential to the sensitivity of the taste buds, the disposal of carbon dioxide and the maintenance of acid levels in the stomach. Thanks to the work at Grand Forks, a daily quota of zinc needed for health—.0005 ounce (15 milligrams)—was established. But for many trace minerals, healthful allotments remain to be determined. The people at Grand Forks should be among the first to know how much is just right.

Taking the measure of muscle and fat

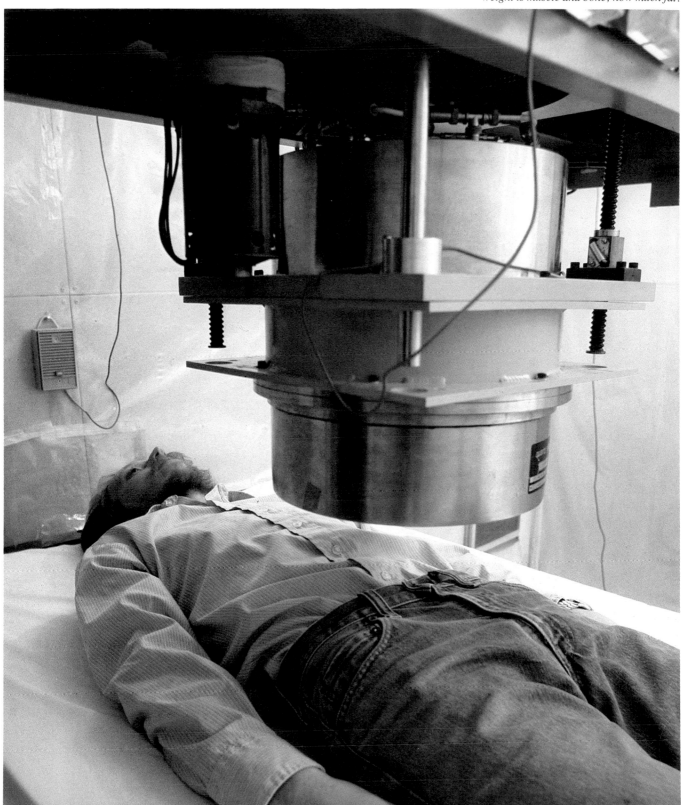

Mike Jackson reclines under a radioactivity scanner, which gauges the potassium-40 in his body. Because potassium-40 is naturally present in all tissue except fat, its concentration shows how much of Mike's weight is muscle and bone, how much fat.

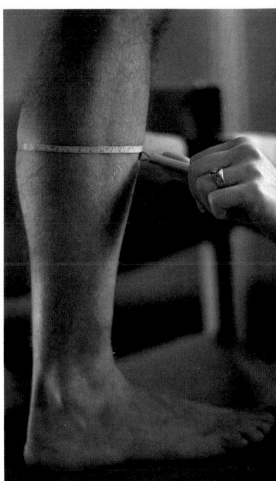

A flexible tape is used to check the circumference of Pat Wolfe's calf and determine whether the experimental diet has changed his muscle size. Calories and exercise are adjusted during the study to keep muscle size from changing, and affecting the body's use of trace minerals.

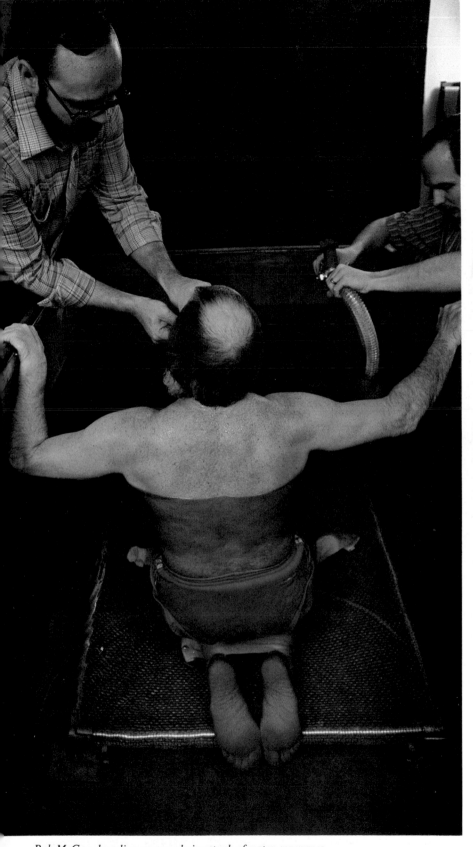

Bob McGee, kneeling on a scale in a tank of water, prepares to receive a breathing tube that will allow him to submerge totally before being weighed. Underwater weighing, which employs the ancient technique of Archimedes to measure specific gravity, is used here to check that the percentage of fat in Bob's body has not altered, and influenced the experiments.

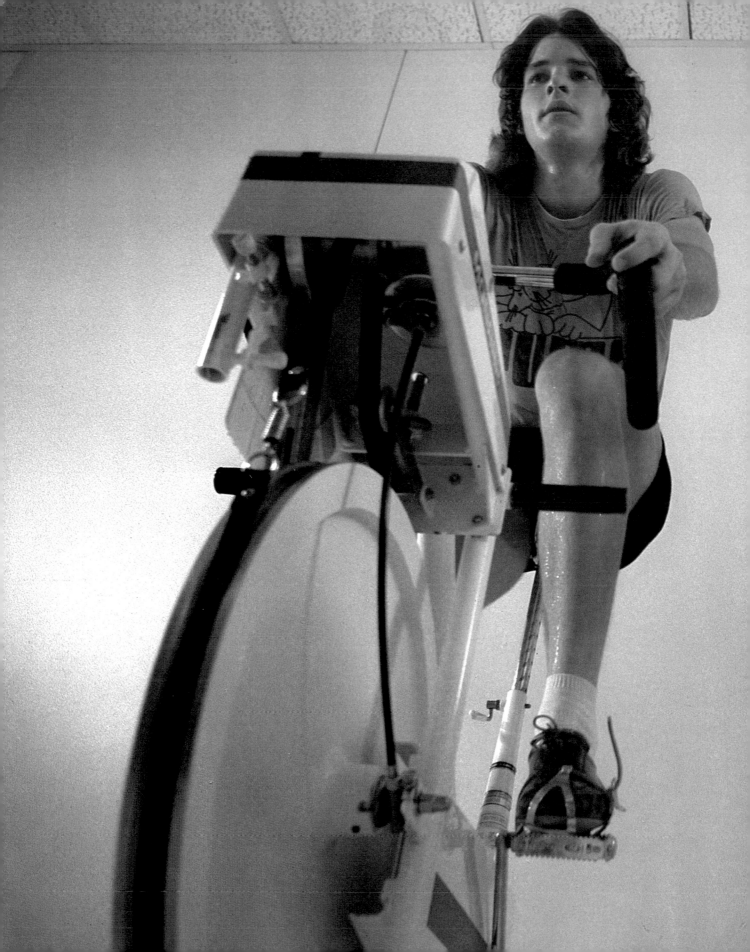

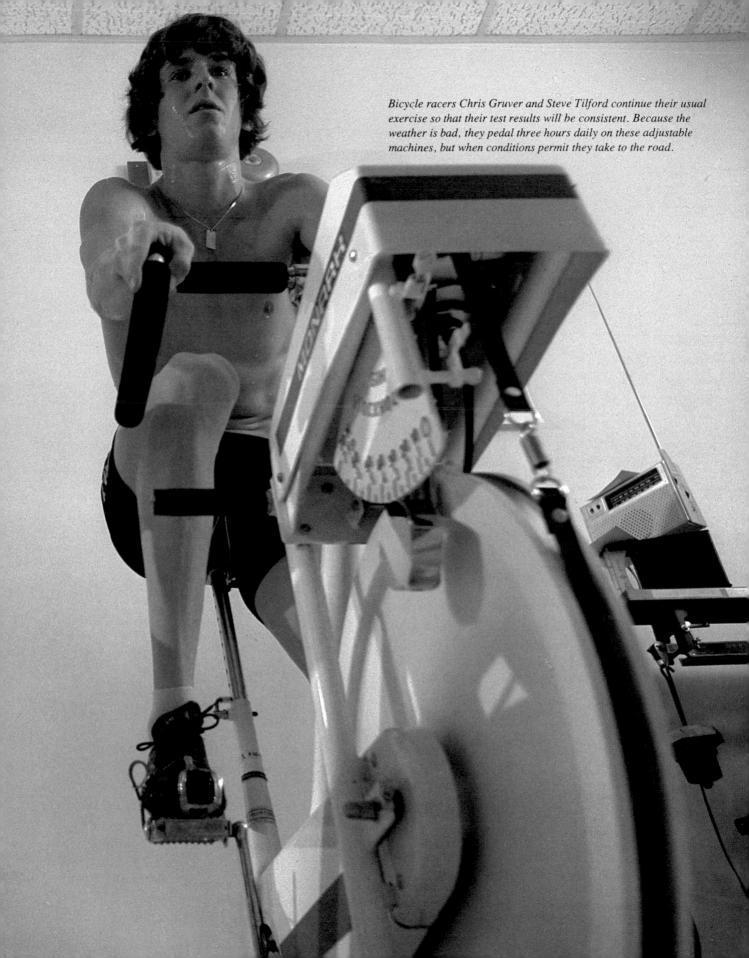

Bicycle racers Chris Gruver and Steve Tilford continue their usual exercise so that their test results will be consistent. Because the weather is bad, they pedal three hours daily on these adjustable machines, but when conditions permit they take to the road.

With chest electrodes wired to a recorder on his belt, Chris begins a 24-hour period in which his heart's electrical activity will be taped. As head nurse Linda Inman looks on, he studies the log he must keep; later the recording is checked for irregularities.

Monitoring the signals from heart and head

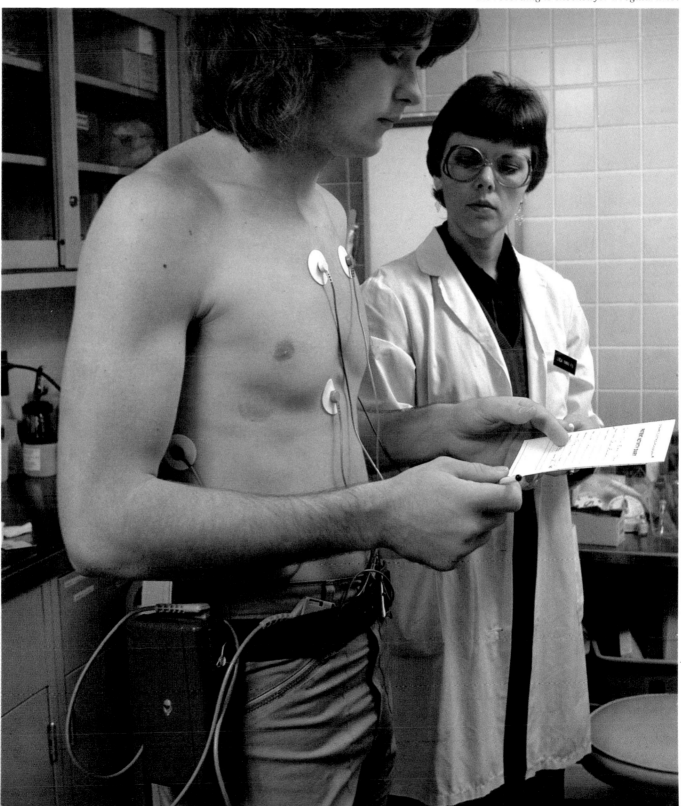

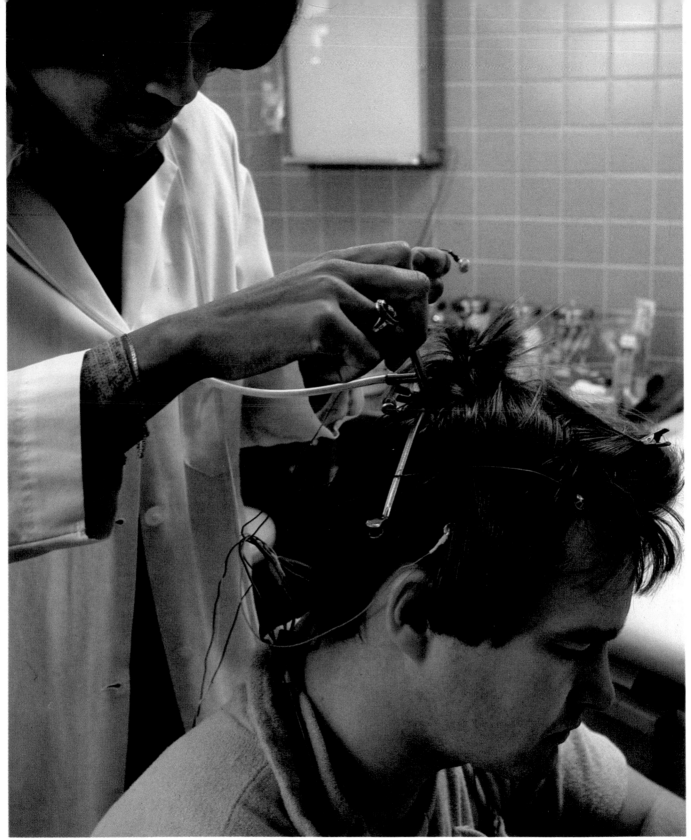

In order to detect subtle alterations in brain function caused by dietary changes, a nurse affixes electrodes to John Blakely's scalp with glue and the special drying device in her hands. The electrodes transmit the brain's electrical signals to a recorder.

Hunting down minerals, even in sweat

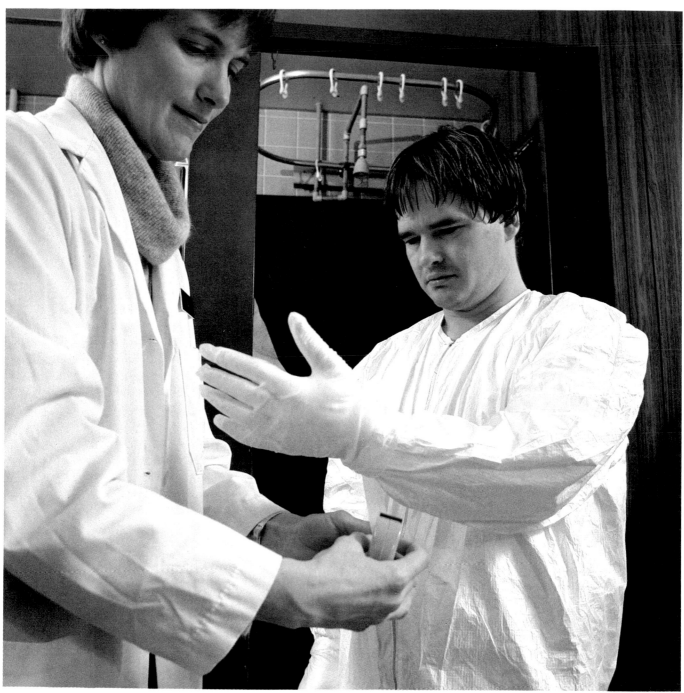

To determine the quantities of trace minerals that are excreted in his perspiration, John suits up for a 24-hour study during which his body sweat will be carefully collected for later analysis. He even wears plastic gloves, sealed with tape, to prevent inadvertent contamination from minerals in the environment.

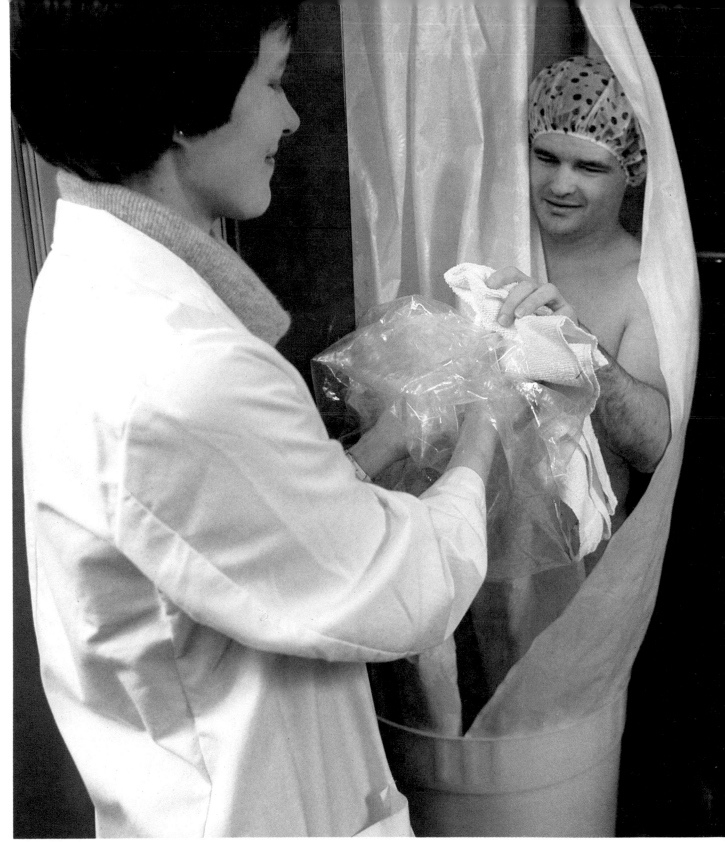

*After 24 hours sealed in his sweat suit, the test subject turns
in his perspiration-filled garment and takes a shower in
distilled water. His shower water is collected in the bucket visible
at bottom, plus his clothes and towel, all to be assayed for the
minerals they picked up from his perspiration.*

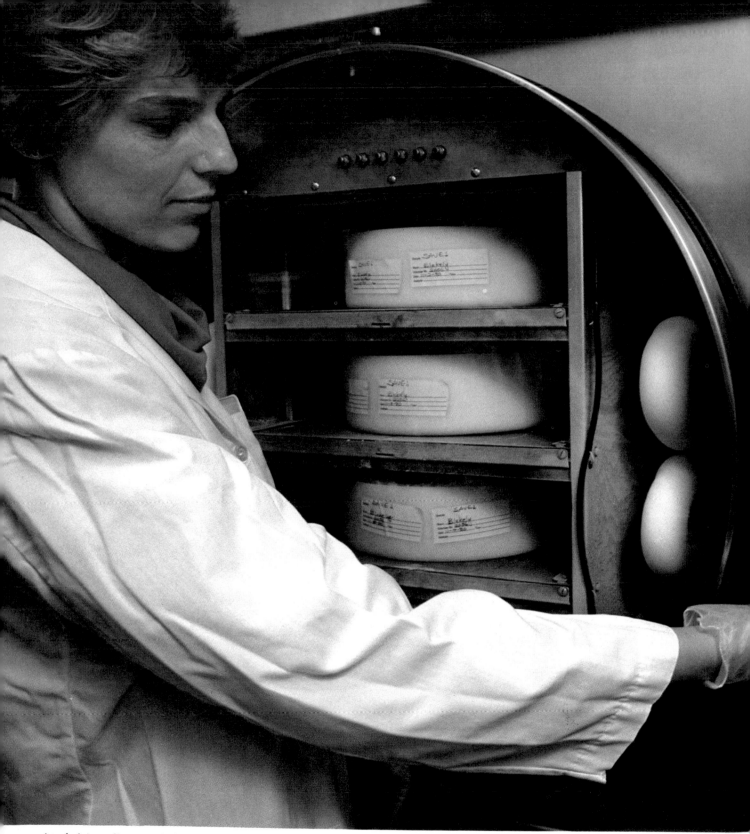

A technician adjusts a unit that freezes samples—shown on the shelves at left—for analysis. Food samples, and the feces and urine collected over a six-day period from each subject and stored here, are then assayed to reveal how much of each of the ingested minerals the body excretes unused and what it retains.

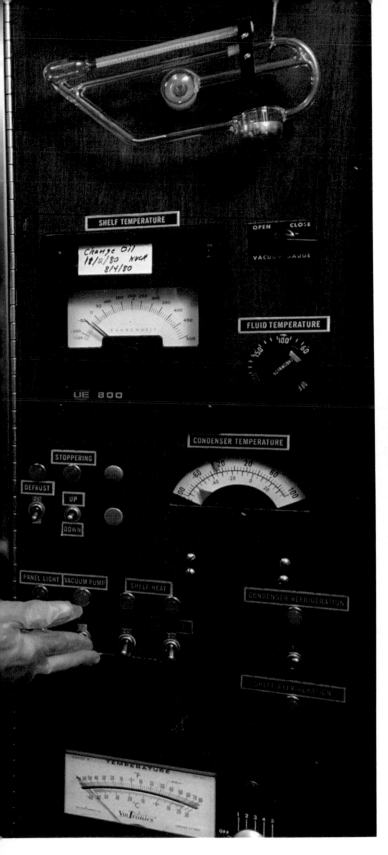

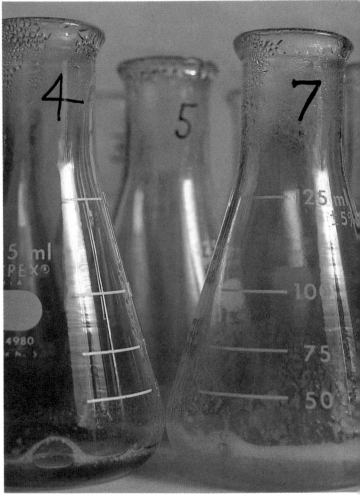

To determine the amounts of minerals present in a test diet, food samples from the duplicate, uneaten portion are combined in flasks with acids similar to the stomach's digestive chemicals and analyzed electronically. This technique detects as little as one part of trace mineral per million parts of other substances.

How to take weight off and keep it off

A wholesome diet not only supplies the right balance of nutrients. It also helps the human body establish a healthy weight—neither too fat nor too thin—and to maintain that weight through the adult years. This ought to be a simple matter, yet it is a major problem in life for millions of people around the world.

In some places the problem is too little weight; tragic undernourishment persists in many nations, as it did until this century nearly all over the world. In the past only the privileged few worried about excess weight. But in industrialized countries today, where food is abundant and technology advanced, a great many people are too fat because they eat more food than they work off. The average Italian, for example, consumes 30 per cent more calories each day than needed. Two separate surveys indicated that about half the population of England is significantly overweight, and in West Germany almost every third person is too heavy. One authority estimated that more than 10 per cent of American children were overweight.

The remedy for excess weight was recognized long ago. A physician of the Second Century A.D., Soranus of Ephesus, recommended the restraint of "excessive nourishment," and also noted the need for exercise. In the 18 centuries that have passed since then, no one has found a simpler solution for shedding excess fat; eating less and exercising more remain the basis for all reducing plans that work. But medical research has come to a fuller understanding of the dangers of obesity, and of its causes.

Although food is the source of obesity, many people who are fat eat sparingly, and many who are thin consume huge meals. Genetics is involved; in addition, infant feedings may leave an individual permanently prone to obesity; and psychological and emotional effects have a powerful impact on body weight. This new knowledge of causes leads to ways to get around the difficulties of eliminating excess fat and thus avoiding its ill effects.

Some body fat is essential. The body of the average healthy young man is 15 per cent fat, of the average healthy young woman 25 per cent. Properly called adipose, fat is a type of connective tissue that serves the functions of insulating, cushioning and lubricating the anatomy; but most important, it stores fuel. This fuel is derived from food, and only some of it circulates through the bloodstream for immediate use. Part of the rest is put aside in the liver and muscles. But the greater portion of the fuel that is not required immediately is converted into droplets of fat, which fill the centers of the fat cells, pushing the other functioning parts of the cells out to the periphery. Between meals, as fuel supplies in the bloodstream and liver begin to run low, the fat in the fat cells is summoned forth and used. After several hours without taking in any food, the body may be supplying more than half its energy requirements from such fat. Ordinarily the loss is promptly made up at the next meal.

But an excess of fat—surrounding the intestines, the kidneys, the heart and other organs, clustering between muscles, lining the abdomen, padding the entire body—is now

The eating preferences of Jack Sprat and his wife are only partly responsible for their contrasting figures, depicted in this 1913 illustration by the English artist Arthur Rackham— heredity, upbringing and stress may also make people fat or thin.

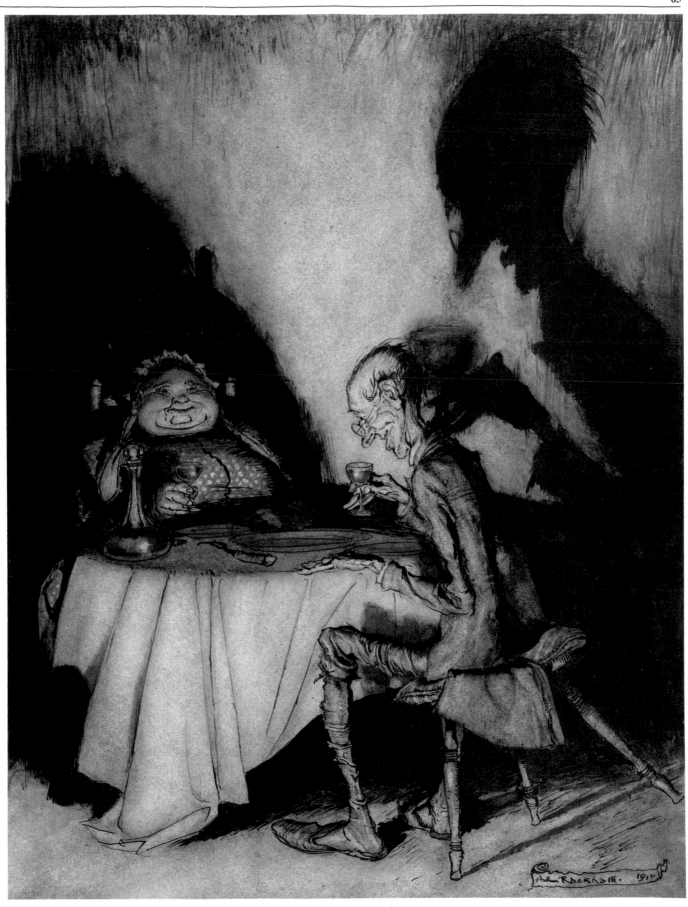

believed to increase the likelihood of contracting a variety of serious ailments. A report of Britain's Medical Research Council began with the flat statement, ''We are unanimous in our belief that obesity is a hazard to health and a detriment to well-being.''

Each added pound must be supported by 15 to 25 miles of blood vessels. The heart must work harder pumping blood to the extra flesh. The flesh itself must be carried around wherever its owner goes, putting a strain on joints and back and rendering most exercise a burdensome task. The obese are more accident prone. They face greater danger when surgery is needed. Above all they may be more subject to diabetes, high blood pressure, gall bladder disease and gout; and there is now a well-accepted association between obesity and certain cancers, notably cancer of the lining of the womb. Obese people, it is all too clear, pay a high price for their unwanted cargo.

The true villain in these health troubles is fat, not weight. The distinction is an important one. Even though overweight has come to be equated with obesity—the medical condition that is characterized by excessive bodily fat—the terms are not synonymous. Yet ever since the first weight-height table, prepared for the Association of Life Insurance Medical Directors and the Actuarial Society of America, was published in 1912, what is considered obese has usually been measured in pounds compared to height instead of being measured as a percentage of body fat. How helpful these tables really are is questionable. As the rotund comedian Buddy Hackett once observed, ''I was reading one of those weight-and-height charts, and I discovered something: I'm not too fat. I'm too short.''

Buddy Hackett's comment contains as much truth as humor. The tables can be misleading. Although too much weight usually means too much fat, it is perfectly possible to weigh a great deal and be lean rather than fat—professional athletes and many construction workers have little fat on their frames but considerable muscle mass, and many of them are overweight according to the tables. These people are not fat. Even more people who do meet the requirements of the tables *are* too fat.

The tables list ''desirable'' weights for various heights. What is considered desirable is found by examining mortality statistics in which people who die are classified by weight; the weight with the lowest death rate is desirable. However, the published tables indicate that variations of 10 per cent from the desirable weight are normal. This scheme gives ranges of acceptable weights so broad they are difficult to interpret. For a height that calls for 150 pounds, the acceptable range covers about 30 pounds. Only someone who is extremely overweight (or underweight) could diagnose their condition from such a table.

More important, the exact relationship between higher-than-desirable weight and health remains in dispute. The Medical Research Council of Great Britain, after emphasizing the hazards of obesity, admitted: ''It is difficult to document the importance of obesity statistically.'' The famous Seven Countries study of heart disease, conducted by Ancel Keys of the University of Minnesota, could establish no direct connection to weight. And a study of utility company employees in Chicago found that men who weighed 25 to 35 per cent more than is desirable lived longer than those closer to desirable weight.

On the other hand, there are other statistics that do indicate danger from excess weight. Life-insurance figures—which are biased somewhat because the data cover only the select groups who buy individual policies—show that overweight people suffer a variety of illnesses and die early. This overall conclusion is confirmed by one of the most ambitious investigations of human health ever made, the Heart Disease Epidemiology Study, which in 1948 began to monitor the physical condition of 5,127 people in Framingham, Massachusetts, a suburb of Boston. Results of the Framingham study showed that the risk of sudden death from a heart attack tripled if a person's weight was 20 per cent greater than the desirable level.

These results, whether they confirm or question the dangers of obesity, are based on measurements of weight, not of fat. Although all authorities insist that fat is the crucial factor, few investigators have attempted to compile health data based on measurements of fat—weight is simple to gauge precisely, whereas fat is much more difficult.

The only precise methods for measuring fat, such as underwater weighing and potassium-counting *(pages 54-55)*, require laboratory equipment. Somewhat simpler techniques use mathematical formulas to convert body measurements into percentages of fat. Much easier is the so-called pinch test, in which a fold of skin in the abdomen is pinched firmly together and its thickness measured. It gives an indication that is rough but may be more meaningful than weight: A pinch of more than an inch in an adult generally signifies too much fat. But the simplest and possibly most useful test is the one employed by nearly all physicians. They gauge fat with their eyes. Wrote one of the world's foremost authorities on obesity and nutrition, Jean Mayer: "If the patient looks fat, he probably is fat."

No esoteric technique is required to make such a visual test of yourself. Stand naked in front of a mirror and turn slowly. Excess fat generally shows up as a bulging middle—the abdomen and, particularly in women, the buttocks. Fat may also be obvious in a woman's arms and thighs. The appearance of bulges in the vulnerable areas is sufficient warning of presumably unhealthful fat; the bulges should be flattened—without striving for a mistaken ideal of unnatural thinness. Some teenage girls and young women who are not fat endanger their health by starving themselves to achieve figures that they consider fashionable *(right)*.

If detecting excess fat is easy, getting rid of it is not. Obesity is quite a bit easier to prevent than it is to correct. It can originate in any of a number of ways—new ones continue to be discovered by researchers—and some of the causes are beyond individual control. Understanding them, however, can help to counter them.

Born to be fat? Or brought up to be fat?

Obesity frequently gets its start in childhood—a third of all cases begin then—and persists throughout a person's life. The odds that a pudgy 10-year-old will grow into an obese adult are 4 to 1. Whether this early pattern results from heredity or from environment is argued. Fat parents tend to beget fat children and thin parents thin ones, but no one knows, as

Too skinny in the midst of plenty

In the industrialized world, only a few people suffer from the other weight problem: too little fat. Most of them are recovering from illness, are unable for psychological reasons to eat enough—or are misguidedly aping a fashion for scrawniness. Checking weight against a standard table of averages, although often a misleading clue to obesity, is a useful guide in this case; anyone who is 10 or more per cent lighter than the average for his height and build—and looks too thin—probably has so little fat he risks his health.

At one time, animal tests were thought to indicate that thin people lived longer than the average. However, recent analyses comparing death rates among those with different body types demonstrate that being underweight confers no advantage in life expectancy—and may be a disadvantage. Lack of fat increases susceptibility to illness, slows recovery and brings on fatigue quickly. It poses a special threat to young women, who may become infertile if undernutrition triggers hormonal changes that unbalance the reproductive system.

More serious is the self-induced starvation called anorexia nervosa, which afflicts many well-off young people, nearly all of them female, between the ages of 11 and 24. Although the condition is marked by absence of appetite, Dr. Hilde Bruch, an authority on the illness, suggested that the symptoms are paradoxical: "These youngsters are frantically preoccupied with food and eating but consider self-denial and discipline the highest virtue." Some waste away to death.

Putting on fat requires the same high-calorie foods many people try to resist: creamed soups, nuts, breakfast meats, and plenty of desserts, piled high with whipped cream or ice cream, in addition to large portions of foods high in carbohydrates and proteins. But the prescription for exercise is the same as for those who want to lose weight. Increased activity stimulates appetite—for some reason only among the thin, not the fat—and helps muscles develop in pace with fat cells.

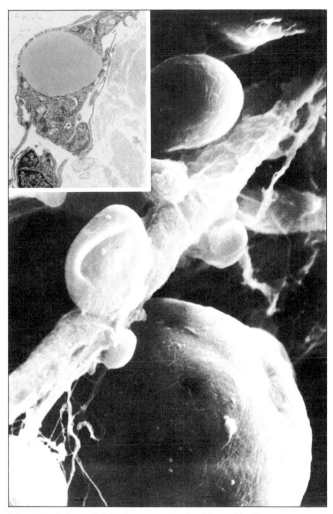

Magnified about 4,300 times, a spherical fat cell—from a rat, but little different from human cells—looms beneath a strand of a blood capillary. The inset, a cross section of a similar cell magnified 520 times, reveals the contents—notably a large droplet of fat that the cell has absorbed, to be stored until needed to meet energy demands. When more fat is eaten than is burned up in activity, such stores build into obesity.

Terryl Foch of the University of Colorado expressed it, whether this is due to shared genes or to shared meals. If meals matter most, then children ought to resemble their mothers more than they do their fathers, for mothers have traditionally done the cooking. Yet scientists have found this is not the case. On the other hand, if it is genes that make the biggest difference, then there is no reason why fat people should tend to have fat pets; yet they do, as other scientists have discovered.

The influence of heredity is suggested by characteristics shared among children who are prone to obesity. Most have short, broad hands and feet and generally rounded conformations. They are larger all over—bigger-boned and more heavily muscled than average for their age. In later years their fat tissue is distributed quite evenly over the body, not centered in the trunk as it is in most people who are not fat as children but become obese in adulthood. Moreover, at an early age the bodies of many fat babies manufacture fat cells that are not only larger but more numerous than the fat cells of leaner children—a finding that may well prove to be the Rosetta stone that reveals the reasons behind lifelong weight problems.

In 1959, Per Bjurulf of the University of Lund, Sweden, examined samples of fat tissue taken from the bodies of 110 men after they had died, and he made a surprising discovery: The fat men had not only larger fat cells but more of them than the thin men had. Bjurulf speculated that the reasons for the greater number of fat cells were probably hereditary. The Bjurulf report was followed by a stream of research on the relationship between hypertrophic obesity (with fat cells that are too big) and hyperplastic obesity (with fat cells that are too abundant).

In one study, a team headed by Dr. Jerome Knittle at the Rockefeller University in New York City overfed some rats while underfeeding others. The team found that the number of fat cells in each animal became fixed when the rat was young—10 to 15 weeks old. And the number of cells depended on how much they ate. Rats that were underfed during the first weeks after birth developed few fat cells and remained lean, with a low fat-cell count, for the rest of their lives—regardless of how much they ate later. The opposite was also true. The overfed rats developed many fat cells and got fatter than the others; these characteristics were unaffected by later changes in diet.

Experiments that were being performed with human beings at approximately the same time yielded similar results. The severest forms of obesity seemed to be caused by excessive increases in the number of fat cells, a multiplication that took place only during certain critical periods early in life. Perhaps, scientists thought, obesity could be conquered if babies and children were kept thin.

More accurate cell-counting techniques, however, indicated that fat cells can increase at almost any time, given sufficient impetus. Still, they proliferate naturally and most extensively in childhood.

One study of children's fat cells, undertaken at New York City's Mount Sinai Hospital, revealed a pattern of variation in both the number and the size of fat cells. The cells grow in size and number until the baby is about 12 months old, when the size of the fat cells is approximately equal to that of an adult. At this point the cells begin to decrease in size (not in number)—but only in babies who are of normal proportions. In these children cell size and number level off at the age of two and remain quite stable until around the age of 10, when both size and number begin to increase again; the increase continues until adulthood.

Obese children never experience either the drop in cell size at one year or the two-to-10 plateau. Their cells continue to swell and multiply throughout childhood and adolescence. By the age of 19 they possess, on the average, fat cells twice as numerous as those of their trimmer counterparts and 30 to 40 per cent larger.

Heredity influences these childhood effects, but overeating plays a big part, too. Experiments on rats at the Rockefeller University demonstrated that fat cells first expand in an attempt to accommodate surplus calories; then, when the cells reach their maximum girth, they simultaneously decrease in size and increase in number—the body builds new storage tanks when the old ones are filled up. An increase in cell diameter may be all that is required to trigger the multiplication of cells. But it is suspected that the total proportion of fat on the body also plays a part: In children, when fat exceeds 25 per cent of body weight, the number of fat cells rises dramatically.

Thus limiting the overall number of fat cells, whether in childhood or later, is a critical factor in controlling obesity. Any increase is permanent and irreversible. If a rat that has been allowed to become obese through overfeeding is put onto a normal diet for a while and then is returned to a high-calorie regimen, the rat will eat more and gain weight faster than it did the first time around. Similar kinds of difficulties plague human beings who harbor too many fat cells. When they go on a diet, the plump people do not slim down as much as other people, even though their individual fat cells may be reduced to normal size.

For these reasons, preventing obesity early in childhood can go a long way toward preventing obesity later in life, particularly if one or both parents or several other close relatives are obese. From birth, the surest way to feed an infant only what is needed for good nutrition is to follow the baby's lead. Most babies know when they are hungry. "If they are offered more food than they need," baby-care authority Dr. Benjamin Spock pointed out, "they refuse it. If they are given less, they show their hunger by waking earlier before feedings and eating their fists."

Because babies must gain weight steadily, it is not easy to distinguish healthy growth from oncoming obesity. Explained the London-based child development specialist Penelope Leach, "Faces are often very round and tummies almost always stick out. If you think your child is getting too fat, look at the upper arms and at the thighs. If there are rolls of fat in those areas, so that the sleeves and the legs of the clothes strain tightly around them, then the child probably is too fat."

The many causes of middle-age spread

Excess fat in childhood, for all the difficulties it causes so many people later in life, still accounts for less than half the world's cases of obesity. Most fat adults were lean children. Men are apt to put on weight between the ages of 20 and 30.

Women—whose bodies naturally acquire more fat than men's, mostly because of the influence of hormones—tend to continue gaining weight into their fifties, often in spurts in response to physiological events such as pregnancy and menopause. In general, both men and women gain by increasing the size of their fat cells rather than the number. Their appetites may not diminish as they enter adulthood, but there is a decrease in how much food their bodies need. They require no additional tissue, for their years of growth are past. Most of them, spending their days behind a desk, get less exercise than they did in earlier years. Simultaneously, the fundamental demand for food energy is reduced by a decline in the basal metabolic rate—the speed with which the body expends calories on such fundamental functions as breathing and heartbeat.

The process of aging also plays another trick on the adult physique, by converting more food into fat than it did in earlier years. Hormonal changes may be involved, but the principal reason is lack of activity. Thus, simply maintaining the same weight year after year does not prevent a gain in fat. In order to stay in shape as the years go by, a person has to increase exercise while eating only enough to hold to the earlier weight.

At one time the thyroid, the metabolism-regulating gland located in the neck, took the blame for the bodily changes that brought on many cases of obesity. Today many other organs and a number of chemicals are known to be involved. One of these is the master substance of metabolism, insulin, which pours into the bloodstream after a meal is eaten to ease the passage of nutrients into the cells, where they are used for construction and repair of body tissues, burned for fuel or put into storage as fat. Insulin, together with the female hormone estrogen, causes more fatty tissue to deposit on feminine frames at the time of puberty than on the bodies of young males, whose increased levels of the male hormone testosterone give them more muscle. And a reduced ability of the body to use insulin brings on the serious disease that is so closely associated with obesity, diabetes *(Chapter 4)*. But now science is discovering even more clues to the mysteries of metabolism and obesity—in the brain, which governs appetite, in the hormones that operate these automatic controls, in the enzymes that govern the accumulation of

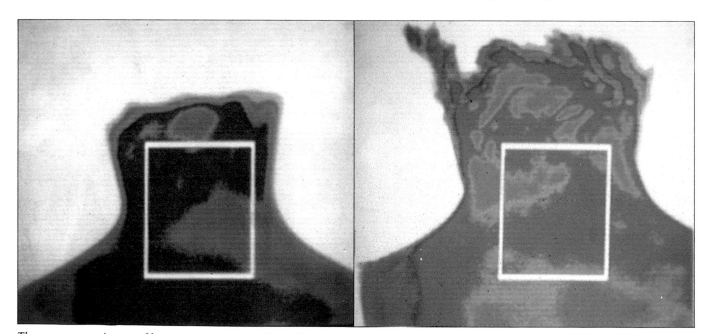

Thermograms—pictures of heat patterns—such as these of a woman's neck gave the first evidence that adults, like babies, have the valuable "brown fat" that may prevent obesity by burning excess calories. This woman's brown fat, indistinguishable above, showed up as turquoise "hot spots" (right) after she took a drug that stimulates brown fat's calorie-consuming action.

fat and even in a "brown fat" that may act to prevent obesity.

Some of the most intriguing research into obesity seeks an understanding of the role of the brain. Somewhere in the nervous system there must be a control—or more likely a set of controls—that keeps weight in balance. Like a thermostat turning the furnace in a house on and off to maintain a steady level of warmth, this "ponderostat" mobilizes a disparate assortment of nervous impulses, cell operations, hormones and enzymes that work in combination to maintain an individual's weight at a set level.

Under certain conditions it is possible for the ponderostat to increase its setting so that the level that is set for an individual's weight is as much as 20 or 30 pounds greater than it used to be. This resetting upward may be triggered by the metabolic slowdown of aging, but it may also occur after a period of overeating and persistent weight gain. An increase in the number of fat cells may have an effect as well.

To control weight, the ponderostat must turn the appetite on or off, thereby helping to determine how many calories are consumed. It must also control the other factor in the fat equation: calorie expenditure.

Responsibility for governing appetite may rest with a part of the lower brain called the hypothalamus. When the supply of nutrients runs low and there is danger of a decrease in weight, the hypothalamus sends out signals that bring on a generalized restless sensation, which gradually grows until the mind takes notice and starts thinking of things to eat. This is hunger. The hypothalamus also has a second message, which it sends out after eating has gone on for a while and there is danger of gaining weight. This neurological signal brings on a feeling of satiety, a warning to stop eating. But the warning can come late. From the time food first enters the stomach, it can take approximately 20 minutes for satiety sensations to develop in the brain. By that time someone who eats rapidly may already have devoured 50 per cent more food than the body needs—this is one of the reasons dieters are urged to eat slowly.

The hypothalamus is made to send out its "eat" and "stop eating" signals by its responses to such influences as levels of insulin and of the energy substance that is controlled by insulin, glucose. It also may be affected by the protein components, amino acids, and by how much total fat the body has previously stored up.

Two of the triggers that turn the hypothalamus on and off are believed to be the hormones beta-endorphin and cholecystokinin. Beta-endorphin comes from the pituitary gland—the growth regulator in the brain—and even small amounts of it can radically increase the appetite. Genetically obese rats have three times the usual amount of beta-endorphin in their blood, and even normal rats will overeat if the substance is injected into their brains. An excess of this hormone is probably involved in some cases of moderate obesity in adults.

On the other hand, it is apparently a deficiency, rather than an excess, of the second hormone, cholecystokinin, that influences obesity. This hormone contributes to a feeling of satiety—when injected into hungry sheep, it made some of them refuse food. Cholecystokinin has been found in both the brain and the digestive tract of humans, and it is deficient in certain obese mice.

Two other substances are also emerging as critical to the efficient conversion of food or fat into energy: the enzyme called sodium-potassium-dependent ATPase and a special kind of tissue called brown fat. Both are active in helping to convert food into energy, preventing the calories from adding to fat stores.

The enzyme causes ATP—adenosine triphosphate, which is the ultimate source of all living energy—to change its chemical form in a way that shuttles sodium and potassium into and out of cells. In so doing, this enzyme uses up between 20 and 50 per cent of the calories in the food eaten. Too little enzyme activity may mean that the calories an obese person receives from even a meager diet are stored as extra fat instead of being burned to fuel cell operation. One study, in 1980, found 20 of 23 obese Bostonians to have substandard levels of the ATPase enzyme in their red blood cells. In a few of the people studied, the enzyme level was found to be as much as 50 per cent below normal.

Brown fat's contribution to weight control comes from the way it dissipates calories from food as heat. This tissue is found in the neck and around the kidneys, adrenal glands and aorta, and it differs from white-fat tissue not only in its color (which actually ranges from yellow to a brownish red), but also in its function. During exposure to cold, the white tissue only insulates but the brown tissue truly warms. It consumes its fat in such a way that fewer calories go into operating the body and more are converted directly into heat. Newborn babies, who are dangerously susceptible to the cold, may have extra amounts of brown fat in their bodies, but as a person grows older the proportion of brown fat diminishes

while the white fat increases. Obese people not only have much more white fat than their less corpulent counterparts, but they may also have brown fat that is not burning up enough calories for heat production.

Even more subtle than the physical influences on fat are those that arise in the mind. Stresses such as anxiety, fatigue, boredom, jealousy, guilt, tension or grief can drive adults and children to overeat. Even frustration or depression about a fat body can have this effect, which naturally only adds to the existing weight problem. There are, in fact, so many

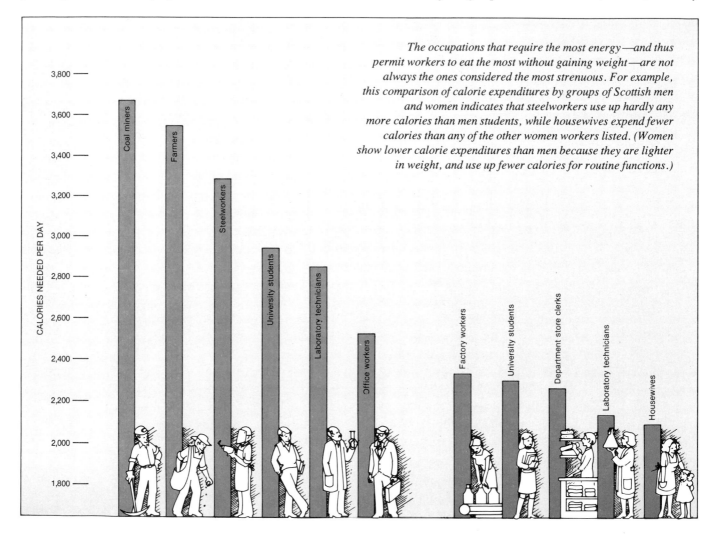

The occupations that require the most energy—and thus permit workers to eat the most without gaining weight—are not always the ones considered the most strenuous. For example, this comparison of calorie expenditures by groups of Scottish men and women indicates that steelworkers use up hardly any more calories than men students, while housewives expend fewer calories than any of the other women workers listed. (Women show lower calorie expenditures than men because they are lighter in weight, and use up fewer calories for routine functions.)

emotions associated with eating and overweight that psychotherapy can help obese people.

Colleen Rand and Dr. Albert Stunkard at the University of Pennsylvania located 72 psychoanalysts who had at least one overweight patient in treatment, and the researchers followed these patients over a period of four years. The patients lost weight slowly at first but more rapidly as treatment proceeded; after four years, most had not regained the pounds shed. Only 6 per cent of these patients had considered weight to be their central problem; the chief complaints were anxiety and depression.

Most people do not need the assistance of specialists to identify emotional distress that may be causing them to overeat. If these people can manage to lessen their stresses—avoiding the source, taking more rest—or at least find some kind of relief besides food for their tensions, they may find it easier to control their weight.

The only formula that works: Eat less, exercise more

The underlying causes of obesity help explain why some people get fat and some do not, and they suggest certain strategies for reducing. For some people, exercise is more important than food in determining obesity. When Mary Louise Johnson and her colleagues at Harvard did research to compare a group of fat schoolgirls with a matching group of lean girls, the obese children were found to exercise less, as might be expected. As might not be expected, however, the fat ones also ate less.

Exercise works in several ways to control fat. The idea that exercise boomerangs by rousing an inordinate craving for food no longer gets much credence. In some fashion not fully understood, exertion generally stabilizes or reduces appetite, possibly by decreasing insulin levels in the blood. In fact, this effect may be most pronounced in the obese. At a Girl Scout camp one summer, the slimmer girls found themselves hungrier than usual because of camp activities. But none of the chubbier youngsters reported an increase in appetite, even though they were equally active, while some of them reported a decrease—and many even lost weight. In another experiment, this one conducted with children who were in

school, it was found that if they had recess before lunch rather than after, they ate less for lunch. Caged laboratory animals are no different: The ones who have exercise wheels eat less than those who spend all their time lying idle.

Among adults, studies indicate that men who exercise are 20 per cent lighter than those who are less active. On women, exercise has an even more pronounced effect. Those who exercise are 30 per cent lighter than their lethargic friends. In addition, exercise can have a helpful psychological effect on people who are dieting. Eating less is, essentially, a negative undertaking. But exercising is doing something, and it can help dieters to feel more positive about their efforts and about themselves.

Any kind of exercise can be helpful in eliminating fat, although such activities as bicycling, running and swimming are generally recommended because they serve to strengthen the body's circulatory system as well. The extra energy that is required for exercise is supplied by the stores of fat in the body. However, exercise by itself reduces weight only slowly. That is why an effective plan for weight reduction requires not only that exercise be increased but also that food intake be decreased.

Going on a diet means going on a kind of budget, except that the aim is not to spend less but to spend more. What you spend is, of course, calories, the measure of the energy-producing value of various foods, and you must spend more than you take in.

A slice of toast spread with a pat of butter, for example, adds about 100 calories to your account; to subtract it again you would have to jog 10 minutes. Similarly, three ginger snaps can be offset by 40 minutes of light office work, and a glass of white wine by an eight-minute swim. Only a negative balance overall will result in weight loss: a loss of about one pound for each 3,500 calories that are spent over and above your intake.

Because exercise withdraws only a little of that stored energy balance, you must also cut down on the calories you deposit to your account when you eat. A man whose eating habits and activities are average and whose weight is stable probably takes in around 2,500 to 3,700 calories a day, a woman around 2,000 to 2,400 calories *(chart, page 72)*. To lose a pound a week the dieter must reduce caloric intake by about 500 calories a day.

Beguiling fads

There is no magic that will accomplish this reduction. There is a whole smorgasbord of ways not to lose weight—with reducing drugs, food substitutes, or the fad diets that provide the fodder for the ever-changing menu at the top of the best-seller lists.

Even the diets that clearly will not work usually have a persuasive rationale. In 1964, a report printed in a German medical journal, *Münchener Medizinische Wöchenschrift,* roused hope and jubilation by asserting that certain foods, because of the labor involved in digesting them, burn more calories than they add; hard-boiled eggs were cited as one example. "Eat, Eat, Eat Your Pounds Away," cried one fashion magazine in an article that said: "If you ate four hard-boiled eggs, you would lose, just because you ate them, 48 calories (equivalent to a 100-yard dash)." Alas, the report was quickly repudiated, and eating as a remedy for obesity was soon abandoned.

Many a person who turns to a fad diet has a history of trying not just one but several of the quick ways to lose weight. Mimi Sheraton, the restaurant editor of *The New York Times,* who confessed in its columns to "an enduring passion for food," tried many diets from childhood on. At age 16, she shed 30 pounds by staying for six months on a low-calorie, high-protein regimen that was intended to be followed only nine days. "That early success was, in a way, my undoing," she wrote, "for I have felt ever since that I can always do it again if I *really* want to."

After having gained back those pounds, she sampled, over the years, a diet of baked potato, butter and nine oranges a day; one of boiled eggs and grapefruit; another relying on hamburger, morning, noon and night; a diet of "a liquid approximating mother's milk"; a rice diet; an ice-cream diet; a weekend of eating nothing but sauerkraut; a "drinking man's diet"; a high-protein, high-fat, low-carbohydrate diet; a fiber diet; and the "last chance" liquid-protein diet. To

quell the rages of hunger, she quaffed grape juice and orange juice laced with unflavored gelatin, she popped diet candies and cellulose crackers and, best of all, she mixed up liquid diet food with chocolate ice cream. The most dramatic way of seeing results, she reported, was to weigh herself on the bathroom scale every night and every morning. "I would register a three-pound loss daily," she rejoiced. "That added up to 21 pounds a week, a figure so encouraging I was moved to celebrate with a victory breakfast of bananas with brown sugar in heavy sweet cream, thickly cut French toast with whipped butter and honey, and a rasher of golden, crisp bacon."

Mimi Sheraton is not alone. Thousands of frustrated dieters have tried fads in their relentless quest for a pleasing reflection in the mirror. And they do lose weight on these regimens—for a while anyway. The popular high-protein, high-fat, low-carbohydrate diets, for example, make it possible for people to take off weight quickly for several reasons. By eliminating carbohydrates—including potato chips, popcorn and cookies—these diets also eliminate a lot of calories. Total intake may amount to only 700 to 1,000 calories a day. Meanwhile, without bread to spread butter on, or potatoes to split and fill with sour cream, the dieter is cutting down on fat as well, even though these diets supposedly include large amounts of it.

Severe restrictions on calories are certain to take off poundage. However, only about 30 per cent of the loss during the first 10 days is fat, according to the report of a team headed by Dr. Theodore Van Itallie of St. Luke's-Roosevelt Hospital Center in New York City. Any diet, balanced or unbalanced, gets rid of the body's carbohydrate stores first, and with the carbohydrate goes water. But the water is quickly gained back when carbohydrates are eventually returned to the diet, as they must be, to prevent a metabolism failure that causes dizziness and nausea.

Low-carbohydrate diets are deficient in vitamin A and the B complex, producing side effects in some people, including constipation, kidney stones, nausea, dizziness, low blood pressure and heart-rhythm disturbances. Nevertheless, these diets remain favorites, even with those who know the haz-

Shaping up in style

One way to lose weight while having fun is to check into a vacation health spa. Most spas offer the pleasures of carefully prepared food, around-the-clock personal service, massages and exotic beauty treatments, but at a premium—a few weeks of such luxurious reducing can cost as much as a new car. For many, however, that is a small price to pay for the posh surroundings and the results: Many dieters lose three to six pounds in a week.

Facilities vary from hearty new recreation complexes with golf courses, tennis courts and Olympic pools, to historic Continental spas with mineral baths, race tracks, opera houses and casinos. The diets are as diverse. At California's Ashram, guests eat spartan vegetarian fare; at The Greenhouse in Texas, elaborately carved vegetables and paper-thin slices of meat are featured.

As little as today's spas have in common with one another, they have even less in common with the fat farms of yesteryear, where wealthy women were pummeled and starved into shape. Today's spas cater to men and women alike, and they stress regular exercise and sensible, if strict, dieting.

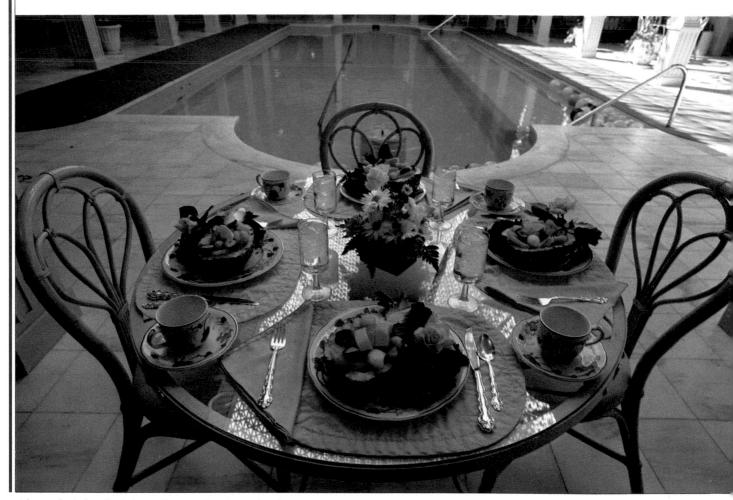

A low-calorie lunch of pineapple, strawberries and melon, heaped into a pineapple shell and garnished with a yellow rose, awaits guests at poolside at The Greenhouse, a luxurious spa in Arlington, Texas. The spa's imaginatively prepared meals are often adorned with decorative but inedible leaves and flowers to satisfy a psychological need for a well-filled plate.

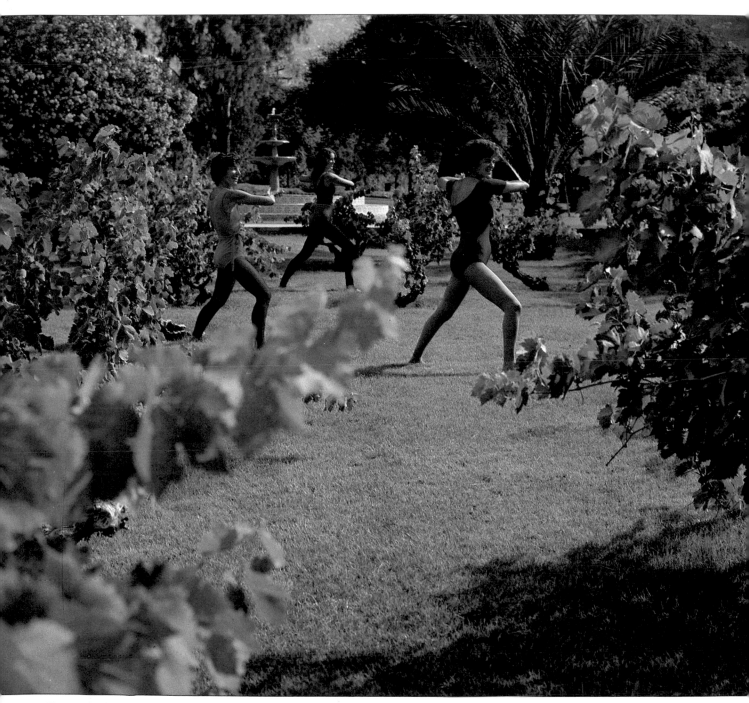

Demonstrating exercises in a garden at Mexico's Rancho La Puerta, encouragingly trim staff members indicate what diet and exercise can do. Guests eat light meals—1,000 calories a day—consisting principally of locally grown fruits, vegetables and grains, and they work off weight with tennis, swimming, calisthenics and hikes through the Sierra Madre foothills.

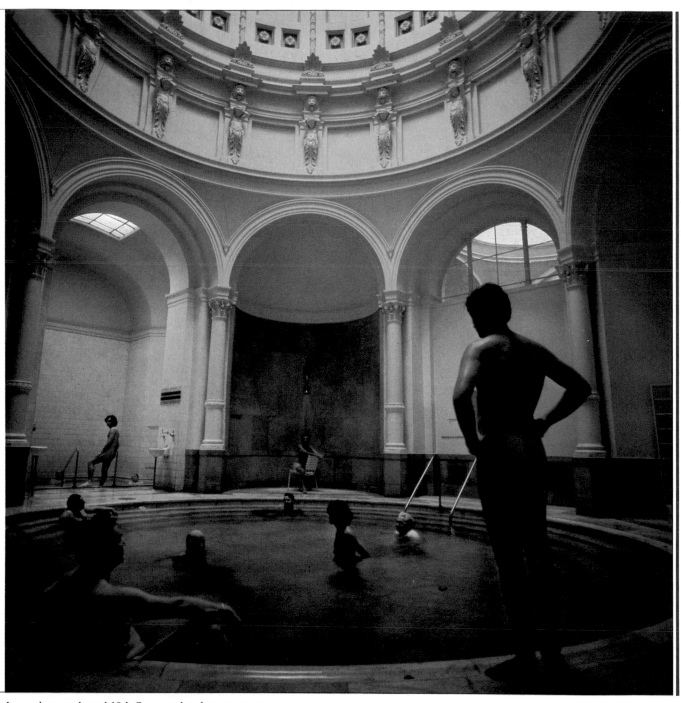

In an elegant, domed 19th Century chamber, guests at Brenner's Park Hotel in the famous German spa of Baden-Baden dip into a pool fed by thermal springs that once soothed the aches and pains of Roman soldiers. Guests at Brenner's Park can complement soaking in the waters with exercise, a strict 1,000-calorie-a-day diet and ventures to the town's gaming tables.

ards. "All I can tell you," said one magazine editor, "is, it's easy, and it's fast, and here I am, down to 125 again." Then she laughed and added, "For the moment."

Equally popular—and hazardous—is the opposite diet: high-carbohydrate, low-protein, low-fat. Calorie consumption can be nearly as low as on the low-carbohydrate diet—approximately 1,300 calories a day. This diet is deficient in iron, calcium, niacin and vitamin A, and of course, protein, threatening the degeneration of muscles. Another troublesome side effect of such a regimen is that defenses against infection are lowered; the body needs proteins to generate protective antibodies.

Both the low-carbohydrate and the high-carbohydrate diets deliver more nourishment than the liquid-protein diet, one of the most restrictive of all regimens. A fast more than a diet—it provides only about 500 calories a day—it is very hazardous. Liquid protein was originally developed by research teams in Boston and Cleveland as a nutritionally balanced mixture for hospital use in treating patients who were dangerously obese. Some varieties that were sold to consumers, however, consist chiefly of collagen or gelatin, both of which are animal by-products lacking certain of the essential amino acids. By 1978, fifty-eight people who had used liquid protein had died. Sixteen of these people—individuals who had no history of previous heart disease—died suddenly of heart failure. Autopsies on some of them revealed heart-muscle deterioration of the kind that is commonly associated with starvation.

For those hoping to lose weight quickly without any kind of diet, there are shelves full of drugs that generally harm more than they help. Appetite suppressants, which are perhaps the most familiar type of over-the-counter diet aid, can temporarily kill hunger, but they can also create physical and psychological dependence and cause high blood pressure, fast heartbeat, dizziness, tremors, hallucinations and, in some instances, impotence.

Other drugs alter bodily mechanisms in order to eliminate weight. The metabolic medications, which speed up the body's burning of calories, can also disrupt the hormone system and cause rapid or irregular heartbeat, as well as headache, diarrhea and fever. Diuretics remove fluid to reduce weight, but in the process they introduce a risk of dehydration. Laxatives speed food on its way through the intestines as a means of limiting nutrient absorption; these not only can cause diarrhea but may damage intestinal muscles and nerves as well.

Tips for taking it off

Drugs and fad diets owe their popularity to the fact that they can reduce weight quickly and fairly easily. They do not work permanently because they do not eliminate much fat unless they are continued over many weeks, and few of them can safely be adhered to for long. Achieving and retaining a healthfully lean figure is not such an easy matter. It demands the self-discipline to make a permanent change in habits of eating and exercising.

To set up a reducing diet for yourself, you must keep some records. The first step is to tally the calories that you take in regularly. Look up the dishes you eat in the tables on pages 160-171, which list calories and nutrients for 290 foods. You may have to adjust the calorie figures listed if you eat portions larger than those indicated—some overweight people grasp the true cause of their condition only on discovering that their customary single portion of sirloin steak weighs eight ounces (880 calories), not the three ounces (330 calories) specified as average. Be meticulous in listing everything you eat: the pastry at a coffee break, an honest total of the number of slices of bread.

From the average sum of daily calories subtract 500 to 1,000 calories, the amount of the reduction depending on how high the existing calorie intake is. The result is the total number of calories in a diet that, in conjunction with exercise, will take away fat gradually and consistently, a few pounds a week. Sharp restrictions on calories are dangerous. Total intake should not be less than 1,500 calories for a man, 1,200 for a woman. The particular foods that make up this diet do not matter much so long as they provide a nutritional balance (a typical day's menu, prepared by the Institute of Human Nutrition at Columbia University, is at right). The simplest scheme is to continue eating the same things you did before but in smaller portions, and cutting down more on the calorie-rich fats and sweets than on other foods. But do not eliminate fats altogether. For health, you need to have a balance of proteins, carbohydrates and fats, as well as a full complement of vitamins and minerals. These requirements are specified in the tables so that you can check the balance of a proposed diet.

Making up a reducing diet is the easy part. Then you have to stick to it until you eliminate excess fat. And thereafter, you cannot abandon it entirely. The caloric content can then be increased, but only enough to maintain the new balance in your body's account. You no longer need a negative balance, withdrawing fat, but you do need a constant balance, with caloric expenditure equal to intake. Otherwise, the lost weight will reappear.

A number of techniques help bolster self-discipline:

• On your refrigerator or kitchen wall hang a calorie chart of the foods you plan to eat most often. Alongside it hang a reminder of your goal, maybe a picture of yourself when you were slimmer.

• Make a careful list of foods for your new menu before you shop, and buy nothing that is not on the list. Also, go food shopping only after—not before—a meal.

• Keep high-calorie foods out of the house or, if this proves a hardship for the rest of the family, at least out of sight.

• In getting a meal together, prepare only the amount of food you plan to eat; do not allow for leftovers.

• Choose foods that require a lot of chewing, such as raw fruits and vegetables; this will help to slow your rate of eating and give your hypothalamus time to send out the signals of satiety.

• Eat at least three meals a day, and do not skip breakfast, even if you just eat lightly. Many overweight people concentrate most of their eating on one big meal—when they are very hungry and consume more than they need. It may be helpful to spread your daily food allowance over a lot of small meals, which help stave off hunger. Laboratory animals that are allowed to eat as often as they like end up with only half as much fat on their bodies as those restricted to two meals a day, even if the total calories consumed are identical.

A Reducing Diet
that tastes good—and works

Breakfast

½ small grapefruit
1 medium egg
1 slice whole-wheat bread, with
1 teaspoon margarine
1½ cups puffed cereal, with
1 cup skim milk
plus as much coffee and
artificial sweetener as desired

Lunch

½ cup tuna (canned in water), with
2 teaspoons mayonnaise
2 slices bread
3 slices tomato, with
1 teaspoon oil
½ cup diced pineapple
plus as much as desired of:
lettuce, pickles, lemon juice, vinegar

Dinner

4 ounces chicken (skinned)
½ cup string beans
½ cup mashed potato, with
2 teaspoons margarine
4 ounces fat-free sherbet
2 dates
plus as much as desired of:
lettuce, radishes, soy sauce, parsley

Snack

1 cup skim milk
1½-inch square spongecake
plus as much coffee as desired

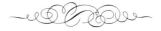

That reducing diets need not be monastic is shown by this menu, adapted from one prepared at Columbia University. It provides 1,500 calories—so little that the average person, with exercise, will lose weight—yet includes a snack and extras. Menus for other days are made up of different foods selected to maintain nutritional and caloric balance (tables, pages 160-171).

• To help your stomach feel full, eat low-calorie foods that are bulky, such as lettuce, cauliflower and broccoli.

The first week of dieting is generally rewarding. The bathroom scale will indicate a gratifying drop in pounds. But then weight loss slows. The slowdown comes about partly because of the way the body initially reacts to the limited intake of calories. It begins by using for energy not so much fat as the reserves of the carbohydrate glycogen. Glycogen is stored with water, and when the glycogen is converted into energy, the water is released, to be excreted. So the first week's big weight loss is mainly water.

After that misleadingly encouraging start, the body consumes more fat than carbohydrate. But a small amount of fat stores a large amount of energy; thus the body gets the energy it needs by burning less fat than it did carbohydrate. Adding to this cause of the reducing slowdown is a little-understood side effect of fat consumption. As the fat tissues are used up, the body somehow begins to store water again, balancing out some of the big weight loss of the first week. Finally, metabolism slows—the body adjusts to the decrease in the supply of calories by using fewer calories.

All these effects interact to make weight loss begin at a gratifyingly rapid rate, then level off to a rate that is frustratingly slow. Yet even the lesser reduction of later weeks can produce impressive effects on your appearance if the diet is combined with an exercise plan. The increased activity influences the quality of diet-induced weight loss, improving muscle tone and firming up slack areas of the body to create a trimmer figure.

The combination of diet and exercise makes spot reducing seem to work, removing bulk from the areas that most people want thinner. This effect has nothing to do with any special kind of fat, such as the ripply, dimpled fat on the hips and thighs sometimes called cellulite. Proponents of the cellulite theory contend that a gel-like substance made up of fat, water and wastes from foods such as ice cream, pork, pastries and alcohol gets trapped in connective tissue. The condition is blamed on everything from poor eating habits to polluted air, and its cure is supposedly a diet low in salt and fat and high in iodine and water, combined with exercise.

Cellulite, according to medical scientists, is simply ordinary fat that is below the skin and is held in place with fibers wrapped around it like strings around a rump roast. As the amount of fat increases, it pushes through these bands, and the problem is compounded with age as the skin gradually loses its elasticity. Such bumpy fat, however, does not call for special kinds of treatment.

No diet, exercise or special machine can remove fat from one particular part of the body. A reducing diet draws on the stores of fat wherever they are—but because they build up mainly around the middle, the middle is the section that loses the most. Exercises that strengthen stomach and leg muscles—as most of the popular types do—pull the reduced tissue mass firm. Thus diet and exercise together will indeed take inches off waist, hips and thighs to create a more youthful shape.

How to keep your figure trim

Because a diet can produce pleasing results in a matter of just a few weeks—a 10-pound loss may reduce the waistline by several inches and fit the body to clothes one size or even two sizes smaller—many people never make the permanent readjustment of their eating and exercise habits that will keep their fat levels under control. They diet for a while and lose weight, and then they resume their previous living style and put the fat back on.

One psychiatrist, Dr. Hilde Bruch, described a patient who thought constantly about her weight and appearance. When she became depressed she would overeat heavily for several weeks, and then all at once she would resolve to get rid of the weight that she had gained. "The dieting usually starts with a big job of housecleaning," wrote Dr. Bruch. "She herself will do the work and feels she does it much better than any cleaning woman would do it; the last thing to be cleaned is the bathroom. Then she takes a bath so that she herself is completely clean and after that the diet begins with three days of complete fasting." Another of Dr. Bruch's patients lost and regained a total of nearly half a ton over a period of 20 years.

Repeated fluctuations in weight impose a severe strain.

The reducing diet, severely limited in calories, need not be continued for a lifetime. But neither can previous habits be reverted to. To live with the new balance of food and activity that will maintain a healthy weight, dieters must modify their behavior. The following techniques for doing so, adapted from those worked out by Richard Stuart at the University of Michigan, are widely used.

The first requires a diary that concentrates on eating behavior rather than simply on caloric intake. It should be started before a diet is undertaken and continued during the period of weight loss. It lists, for every meal or snack every day, exactly what the dieter eats, at what time of day, with whom and in what state of mind. Even though it is a tiresome process, record keeping may be the most valuable part of the behavior-modification program because it helps people to see that they really are eating too much, and it describes the circumstances.

The second step confines eating to an extremely narrow set of conditions. To break old associations, the dieter must eat only at specified times, using only certain utensils and settings—a special place mat with blue fringe, perhaps. Food is eaten in only one location—at a table in a room separate from the kitchen, because in the kitchen the urge to take extras is too easily satisfied. Mealtime is devoted exclusively to eating, unaccompanied by reading or television, so that attention is concentrated on the mealtime, its setting and the food itself—what it tastes like, how it feels as it is chewed and swallowed. A few months of such conditioning brings under control the automatic reach for food when the television is turned on; the desire to eat arises mainly when food is laid out on that mat with the blue fringe on the dinner table. In behavior-modification jargon, this is known as "controlling the stimuli."

Controlling the act of eating itself is step three, and chiefly it consists of slowing the speed at which food is consumed: Count chews; lay down the fork between mouthfuls; follow each swallow with a bit of conversation. This sounds rather silly and artificial, but it helps the conscious mind gain control over the eating process. It also gives the brain time to bring sensations of satiety into play.

The fourth step is a reward for good behavior—not for weight loss itself, because pounds come and go, and often rather unpredictably, but for long-term alterations in habits. Hearty and frequent comments of approval from family and friends provide one effective type of reward. Stuart also recommended a schedule that enables the dieter who follows the required patterns to earn "tokens," which then can be exchanged for specified benefits. A mother with young children who adheres to her diet for two weeks, for example, might be guaranteed three hours of baby-sitting services for the tokens thus acquired.

Such programs of behavior modification are well suited to use by organized groups, which in many cities bring dieters together for mutual assistance. Most people who change from fat to thin, however, do so on their own, at home, using common sense and determination. One who did is Lillian Singer. A schoolteacher, Lillian Singer was 23 years old and had been married just a year when she decided she did not like the way she looked. She began cutting back on sweets, dairy products and bread, and she started to exercise with daily calisthenics. In eight months she shrank two dress sizes to a shape she then retained, with only minor fluctuations, through the years.

She stayed thin without the benefit of special programs, even without a set of scales, guided, she explained, by the way her clothes fitted. When her favorite slacks felt tight, she knew it was time to watch her eating. Nor did she suffer the attacks of hunger that torment so many dieters. "I don't want cookies and cakes, they're too greasy and sweet," she said. "And I miss my exercises if I'm too busy for them. I'm doing what I want to do."

Lillian Singer pointed out that her granddaughter was allowed few fattening foods because of a tendency toward obesity on both sides of the family. The child ate raw vegetables for snacks, was virtually unacquainted with soda and candy, and had never had any milk but skim milk from her early years. "When I was a girl," Lillian Singer recalled, "I drank whole milk with extra cream added to make it richer—that kind of thing was considered healthful then. Now I have a grandchild who's never tasted either of these things." ✻

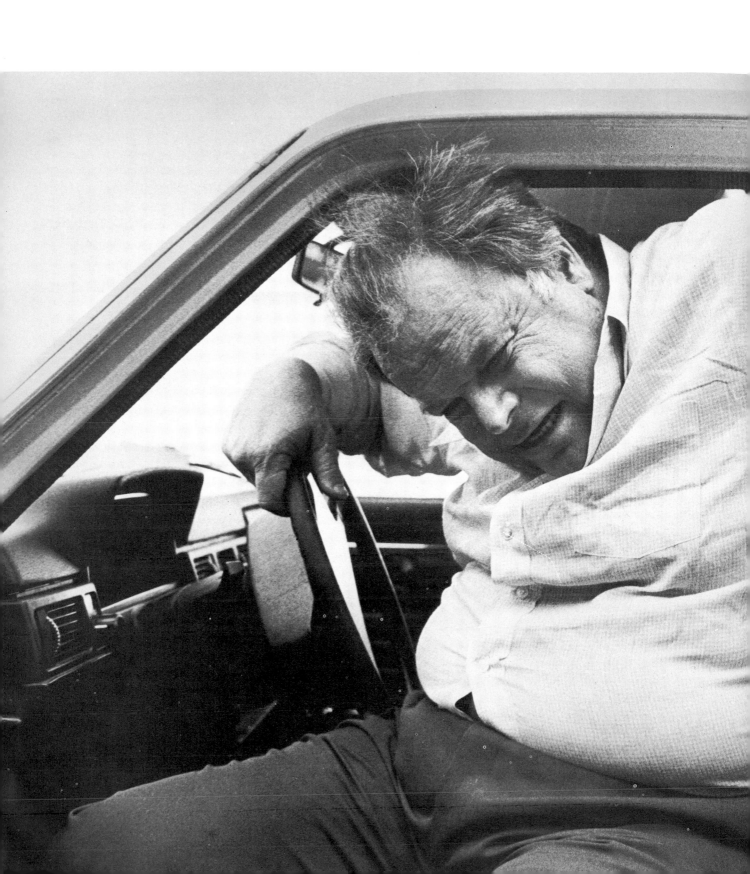

One man's triumph over fat

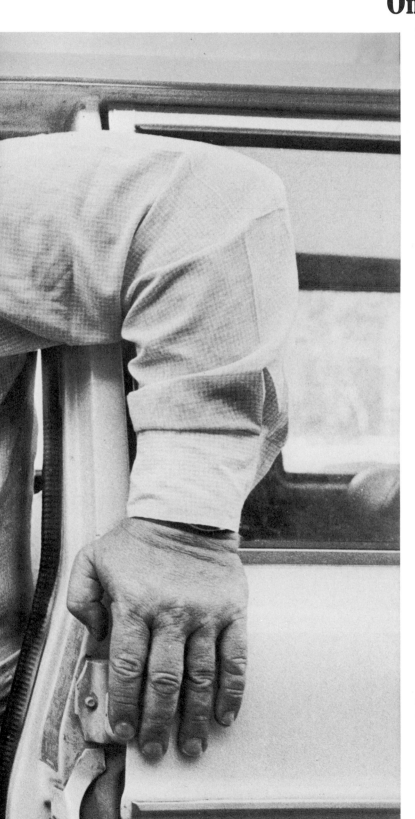

For 305-pound photographer Bob Adelman *(left)*, getting in and out of cars was trouble enough. Flying in cramped airline seats, however, was absolute agony and bending over was next to impossible. When he sat down to tie his shoes he groped over the slopes of his 49-inch chest and the mountain of his 52-inch stomach for the laces and emerged from the ordeal out of breath. "I was happy," he remembered, "because I was eating all the time, but I was a human balloon." In the fall of 1978, he vowed to lose weight.

Adelman had dieted before. "I lost some weight," he said, "but then, like 90 per cent of the people on diets, I relapsed." What he needed was a program that would radically change his eating habits so he could keep lost weight off. He found such a program at the Weight Control Unit of St. Luke's-Roosevelt Hospital Center in Manhattan.

Established in 1977 as a research center to study obesity, the St. Luke's unit accepts only about 200 new patients a year, most of them 70 to 80 pounds overweight. Once accepted, a patient first undergoes a series of psychological and physical examinations. These range from routine intelligence tests, through familiar medical measurements—height, weight, blood pressure and the like—to arcane evaluations requiring complex devices and techniques. Then the reducing begins.

Losing weight at St. Luke's involves more than dieting. "The treatments all include some form of diet," said the program's founder and director, Dr. Theodore B. Van Itallie, but also emphasize what he calls "life rearrangement." Calories are reduced, exercise is increased, and patients are shown how to modify their behavior so that they eat no more than they should *(box, page 86)*.

"The only thing that really helps is to change habits," said Dr. Van Itallie. For Bob Adelman, those changes were profound. But so were the changes in his body.

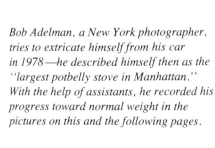

Bob Adelman, a New York photographer, tries to extricate himself from his car in 1978—he described himself then as the "largest potbelly stove in Manhattan." With the help of assistants, he recorded his progress toward normal weight in the pictures on this and the following pages.

Assessing the size of the problem

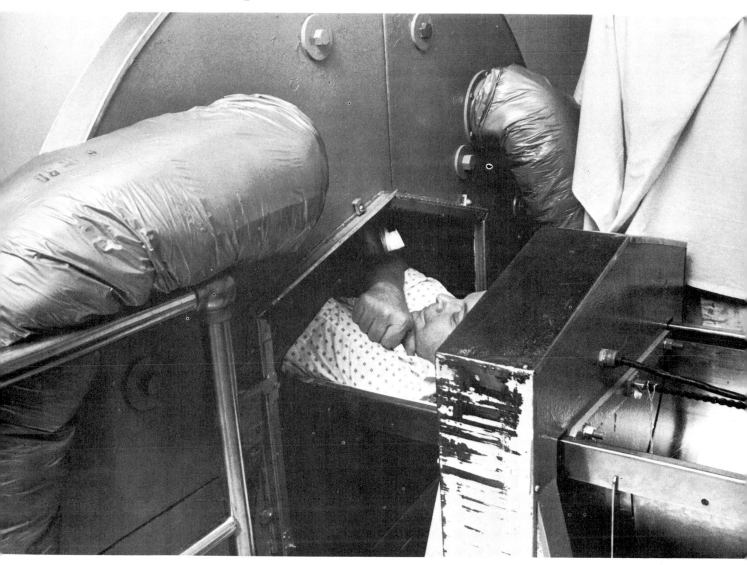

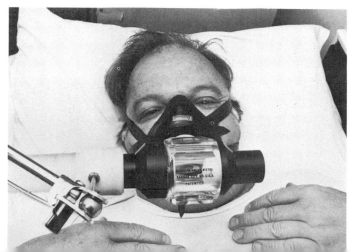

Wedged in a steel cylinder six feet long and 20 inches across, Bob Adelman is about to disappear into a machine called a 4-Pi liquid scintillator whole-body counter. He will reappear about five minutes later, the machine having calculated his body fat: It counts emissions from radioactive potassium, naturally present in the body's lean tissue but virtually absent in fat; by gauging a person's lean tissue, researchers can deduce the amount of his fat.

On his back in a hospital bed, Adelman breathes into a mask connected to a machine that measures his basal metabolism—the amount of energy his body uses at rest. This test, made when Adelman weighed more than 300 pounds, showed that he burned 2,000 calories per day at rest. The figure helped therapists determine a caloric limit that would help him lose weight.

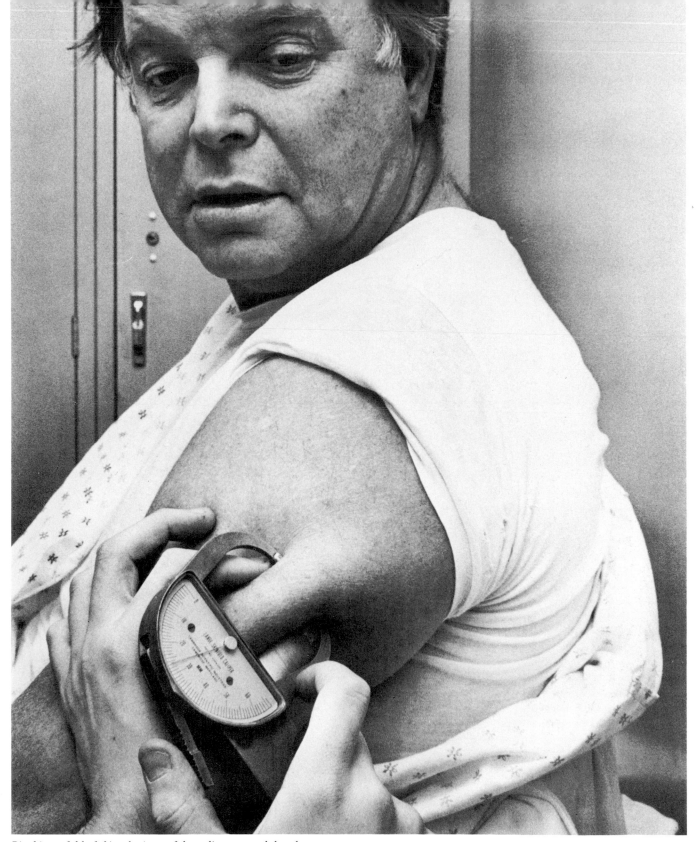

Pinching a fold of skin, the jaws of the calipers reveal that the amount of fat on the back of Adelman's upper arm measures 27 millimeters (about an inch). This measurement, coupled with those from the shoulder, the front of the upper arm, the chest and the abdomen, is taken by staff members at St. Luke's to confirm determinations of fat made by other methods.

Working toward a solution

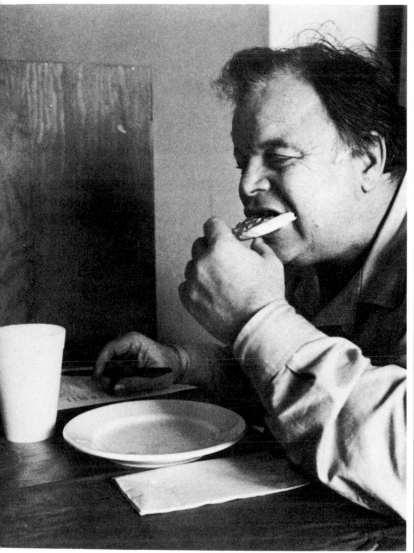

Munching an English muffin that will be washed down with apple juice, Adelman takes part in an eating-behavior study at St. Luke's. After finishing, he was asked to write about the experience—what he ate, when, how much, how long it took, his mood, and an estimate of calories consumed. Adelman found the practice disagreeable: "I hate to write, and, what's more, I was appalled to discover the importance of food in my life."

How to change eating habits

The following tips, adapted from those given participants in the St. Luke's reducing program, explain how to alter food habits—from supermarket to cleanup—to help lose weight.

BUYING FOOD. Plan meals and snacks before shopping, then make a list and stick to it. Shop when you are not hungry. Avoid the aisles with desserts and snacks. Buy small-sized containers or units. Put groceries in the trunk of the car to avoid snacking on the way home.

STORING FOOD. Repackage some foods into individual servings: Cut cheese, for example, into bite-sized pieces and wrap them for a handy snack. Store food out of sight—not in countertop cookie jars or nut bowls—and place it at the rear of cabinets and refrigerators. Store food only in the kitchen or pantry.

PLANNING MEALS. Plan daily food intake, including snacks, and stick to the plan. Schedule all meals and snacks. Write down what you are going to eat and how much; this will make you conscious of the act of eating. At a restaurant, decide before entering which food you will order.

PREPARING FOOD. Prepare food in small amounts, and use foods that demand preparation instead of those that can be eaten straight from the package. Make broiled rather than fried dishes. If you are tempted to snack while you cook, sit down—to heighten your awareness of eating.

SERVING FOOD. Serve meals in the kitchen, not from bowls at the table, so that second helpings are out of reach.

ACCEPTING FOOD. Make a habit of declining food that is offered you. Ask family and friends not to give food as gifts.

EATING FOOD. Delay eating until you are really hungry. Restrict your eating to the dining room. Avoid distracting activities while you eat: You may consume extra food unconsciously if you read or watch television. Eat preferred foods first; that way you are more likely to stop eating when you are full. Eat slowly, putting down your utensils after each bite, and chew thoroughly.

CLEANING UP. Clear the table immediately after eating. Discard or give away tasty, tempting party leftovers.

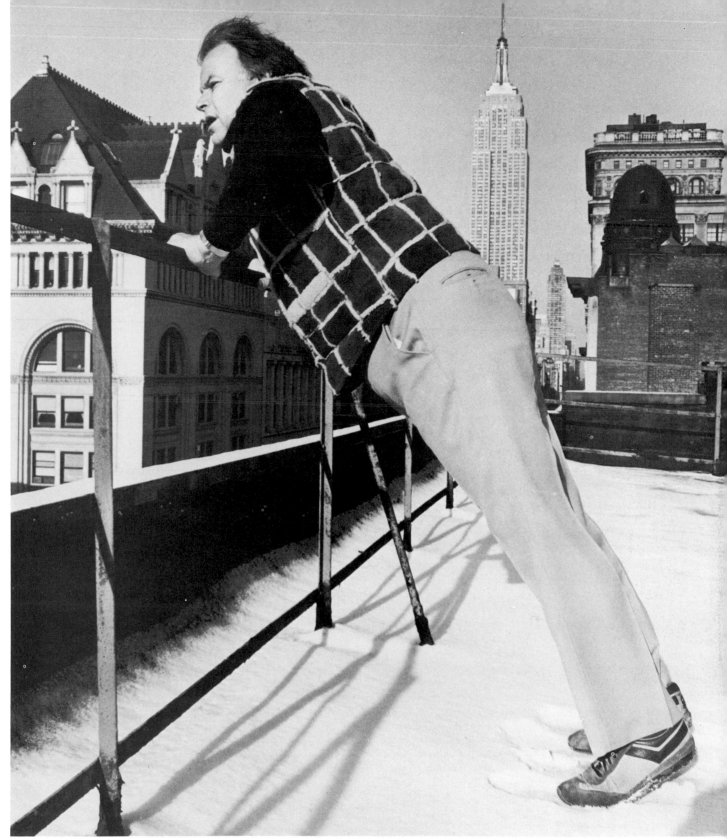

*Huffing and puffing at the railing on the snowy roof of his
Manhattan apartment, Adelman does a modified push-up. At first
his exercise was limited to simple calisthenics such as this;
soon his regimen included more vigorous swimming and jogging.*

Keeping track of lost weight

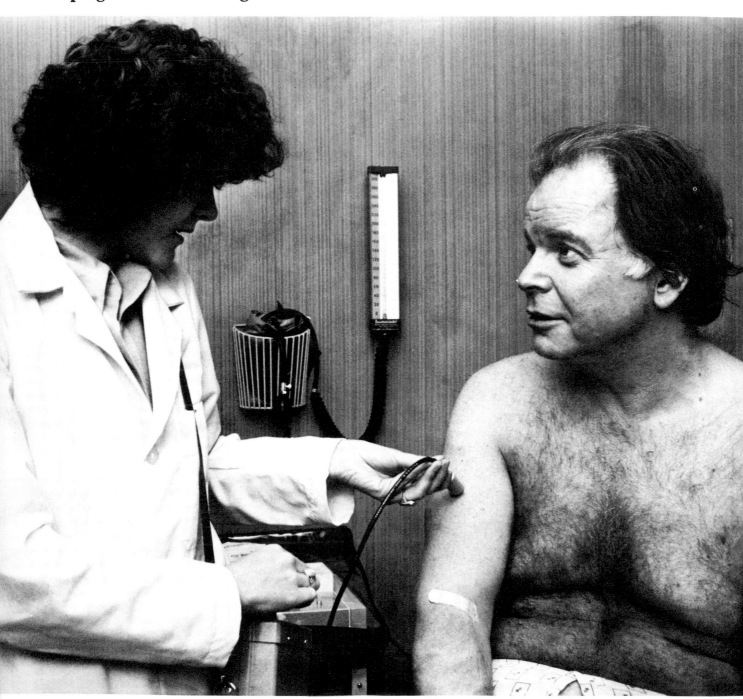

To check on his progress after four months in the St. Luke's
program, Adelman underwent a second round of tests. Above,
a technician applies a special probe to his upper arm to
measure the thickness of his fat. The instrument beams ultrasonic
waves through his skin and into his arm, then analyzes echo
patterns; lean tissue reflects more sound waves than fat does.

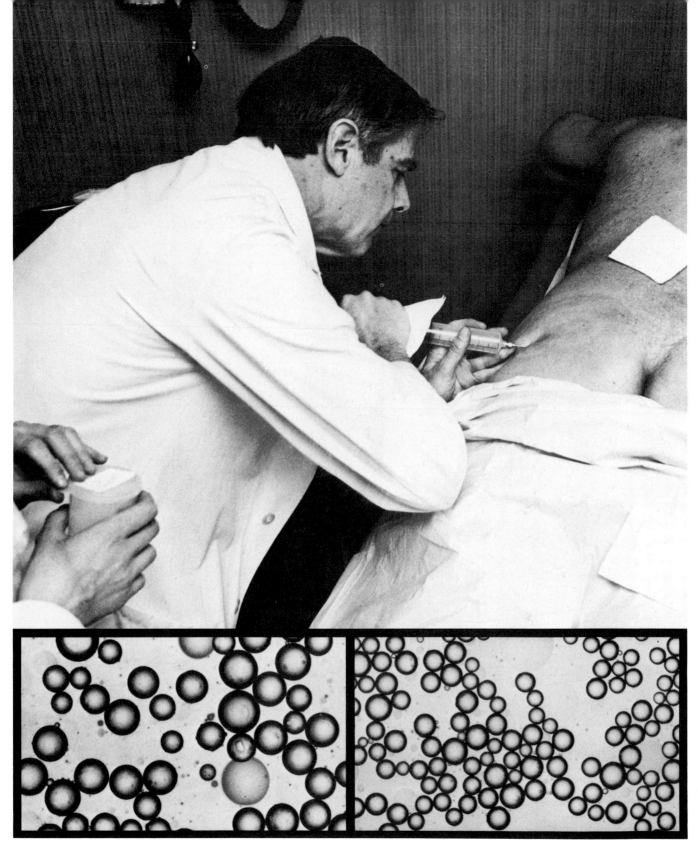

At top, Dr. Van Itallie uses a large hypodermic needle to withdraw fat cells from Adelman's buttocks. This was the second of three such "fat-cell aspirations" Adelman underwent in his first year in the program. Above, the photomicrograph at left shows his fat cells at his 305-pound peak in the fall of 1978; at right, one year later, his fat cells had decreased in size by more than half.

The goal attained: "I'm triumphant"

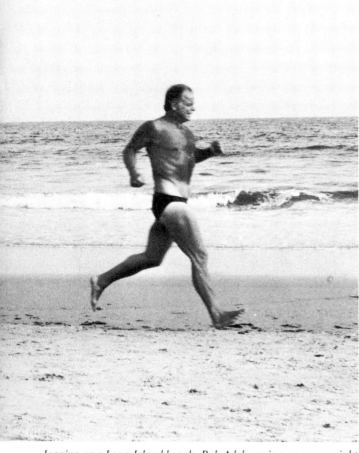

Jogging on a Long Island beach, Bob Adelman is a new man eight months after enrolling in the St. Luke's Weight Control Unit. His weight by then was down to a creditable 190 pounds, his diet a moderate 1,200 to 1,300 calories a day, and he was jogging from 15 to 20 miles a week. "You can see," he said with pride, there was "a strong man under all that fat."

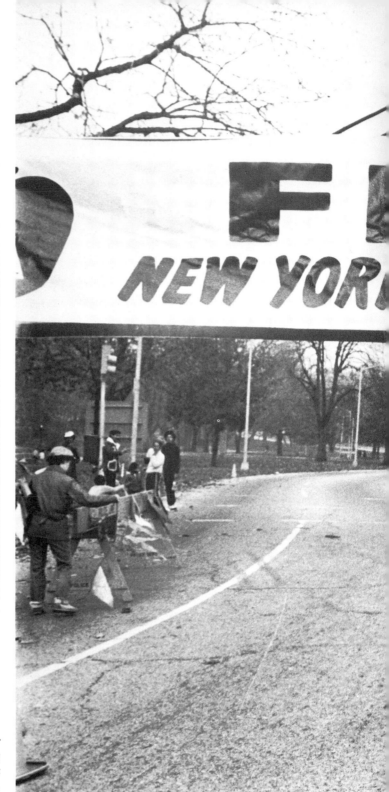

On Thanksgiving Day, 1980, barely a year after starting his program, a beaming Adelman comes to a satisfied halt after a 6-mile race. He had lost 115 pounds. "People don't recognize me," he said. "I have a new disguise—myself. I look like I just hatched out of that 305-pound blob."

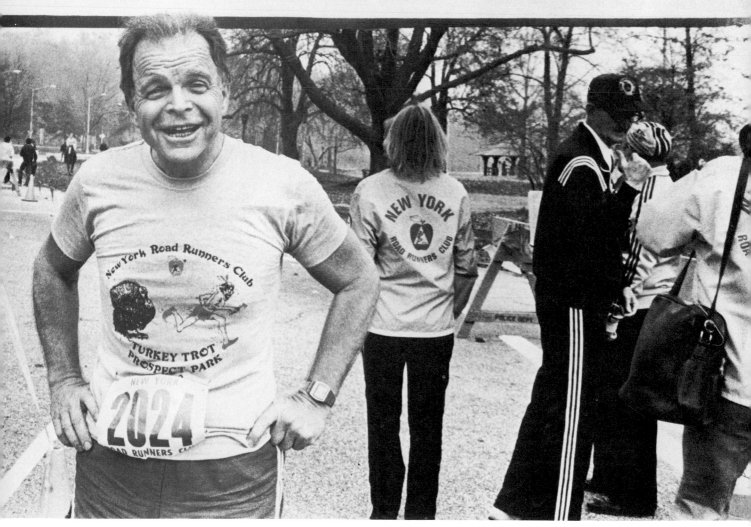

CHAPTER 4

Eating to stay well

The truth about sweets and tooth decay
Why milk makes some people sick
Food allergy: facts and fictions
The elusive cancer connection
The virtues of fiber
Coping with diabetes

From the dawn of history sages have ascribed almost supernatural power to food, alternately blaming it for bodily ills and crediting it with miraculous cures. In the Fourth Century B.C. the Greek physician Hippocrates based his entire scheme of prevention and treatment of disease on food. For more than two thousand years his disciples perpetuated this notion and expanded the list of dangerous foods. In the book *Anatomy of Melancholy,* the 17th Century scholar Robert Burton reviewed the contemporary list of banned foods— and found on it virtually every comestible known. Beef was condemned because it "breeds gross melancholy blood"; pork was "altogether unfit for such as live at ease"; cabbage "causeth troublesome dreams, and sends up black vapours to the brain"; fruits "infect the blood and putrefy it."

Understandably the ancient physicians also relied on supposedly safe foods to cure illness. Hippocrates, maintaining that "thy food shall be thy cure," prescribed virtually every food that he did not prohibit. Dysentery was treated with myrtle, apples, wheat flour, beans, eggs, milk and barley mush. Other authorities prescribed leeks, beans, truffles, celery, pigeons and turtledoves. During the Second Century B.C. Cato the Elder, a Roman statesman, extolled cabbage as a panacea. Although it is easy to scoff at the ancients, a mystical belief in the power of diet has never waned. When cholera ravaged the eastern seaboard of the United States in the 1830s, fruit, salads and uncooked vegetables were blamed, and several cities banned their sale.

Similar myths persist today. Many teenagers are convinced that sweets, particularly chocolates, cause acne. Some soldiers and sailors still assume that their food and drink is laced with saltpeter, which is supposed to reduce the male sex drive; eggs, oysters and truffles, on the other hand, are considered aphrodisiacs. Many food combinations—tomatoes and milk, fish and ice cream, and chocolate and licorice, among others—are believed to interact badly, causing nausea and vomiting if eaten together. Honey and vinegar are touted as a cure for arthritis, fish is widely considered an intelligence-stimulating "brain food" and steak is recommended as a source of strength.

Here and there among those tales are snippets of useful folk wisdom. Cato the Elder was partly right about cabbage, for scurvy was common in ancient Rome, and cabbage contains large amounts of the scurvy cure, vitamin C. The other ideas, however, are fantasies. No particular combinations of foods are especially upsetting—except perhaps psychologically. Nor does chocolate bring on acne, or any single food have much effect one way or the other on intelligence, strength or sexual performance.

Yet there is no doubt that Hippocrates was on the right track. Some foods cause diseases, others prevent or cure them. The extent of the link between diet and disease is fiercely debated by physicians, laboratory scientists and epidemiologists, and the evidence is continually being re-evaluated. A food that is confidently and authoritatively recommended in one decade may be warned against in the next. In spite of these uncertainties, knowledge about some

The foods at right are rich in fibrous materials—chiefly complex, indigestible carbohydrates—that promote healthy digestion. Fiber relieves constipation and prevents colon infection, and some authorities believe it may help prevent intestinal cancer.

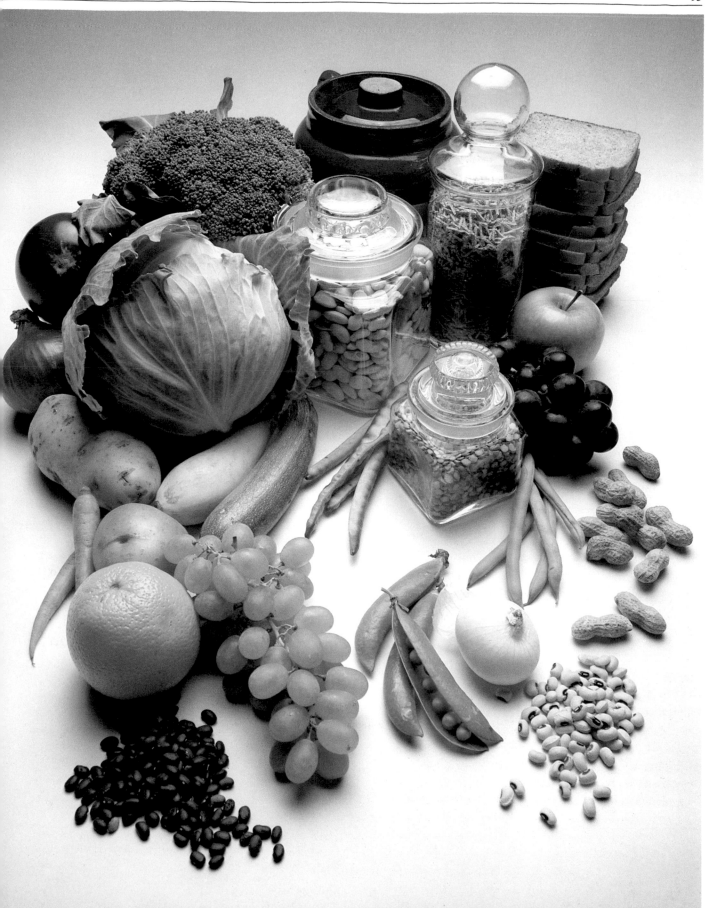

aspects of the diet-disease connection is solid and reliable.

At least three kinds of afflictions, rarely fatal but all very troublesome to large numbers of people, are unquestionably caused by food. Tooth decay, suffered by almost everyone in the world, is known to be intensified by the consumption of sweets. There are also groups of foods that make some people sick to their stomachs. One is milk, which cannot be digested by many older children and adults. In addition, large numbers of people are allergic—or convince themselves that they are—to certain specific foods, reacting to them with the rashes and sneezing commonly associated with dust or pollen allergies.

Mountains of evidence also implicate certain foods as contributors to three major killers: cancer, heart disease and high blood pressure. How much the suspected foods contribute is still being disputed, and disagreements continue about the effects of various foods. But the fact that diet has an influence is undeniable.

All these diseases can be controlled by modest modifications in the kinds and amounts of foods people eat. It is now possible to establish what scientists call a "prudent diet" that could add years to the average life span.

Equally important, diet can be used to treat, and in many cases to cure, a number of diseases that it does not cause— a category that includes such chronic, debilitating disorders as gout, ulcers, acid indigestion, constipation, and the intestinal disorder called diverticulosis. Until recently physicians often prescribed an onerous, unpalatable diet in treating such diseases. But modern research has proved that minor dietary changes—eating more frequently, perhaps, or substituting soothing foods for irritating ones—actually deliver better results.

Finally, diet can be used both to treat and in some cases prevent one unique, enigmatic ailment: diabetes mellitus, the third leading cause of death in industrialized countries, afflicting 5 per cent of their populations. Although heredity plays a part in the two major types of diabetes mellitus, researchers no longer believe that genes are the sole cause. Virus infection, diet and obesity all are important precipitating factors; some scientists argue that obesity alone, without genetic fault, is enough to cause the most common type of diabetes. And in the treatment of diabetes, diet is an essential part of the prescription, either by itself or in conjunction with drugs such as insulin.

The truth about sweets and tooth decay

Of all the connections between food and disease, one that proved especially puzzling is the link between sweets and tooth decay. The hazards of sweet foods were recognized by the ancient Greeks; Aristotle, observing the contemporary passion for figs, asked, "Why do figs, which are soft and sweet, damage the teeth?" After the Persians learned to refine cane sugar into pure crystals in the Fifth Century A.D., Venetian merchants developed a thriving sugar trade—and exacted an exorbitant price in tooth decay as well as money. As late as the 16th Century, Britons paid 25 times as much for a pound of sugar as for a loaf of bread. Those wealthy enough to afford marzipan and sweetmeats soon became martyrs to dental disease. One unkind contemporary described the aging Queen Elizabeth I as having a hooked nose, narrow lips and black teeth, "a defect the English seem prone to from their too great use of sugar."

The consumption of sugar—and the incidence of cavities—has been increasing ever since. Farmers in the Iron Age, for example, probably ate about seven pounds of sugar annually, all of it in fruits and vegetables. In 1900 the average Briton consumed about 80 pounds per year, and only 11 per cent of the 12-year-old children were free of dental cavities. By the 1950s the average sugar consumption was about 100 pounds per year, almost 98 per cent of the 12-year-old children had cavities, and the overall cavity rate was six times that of ancient Anglo-Saxons (as calculated from their skulls). A generation later the per capita consumption of sweeteners in Britain and most Western countries was about 120 pounds a year. In the United States, three quarters of the sugar is now added by food manufacturers—not only in such treats as chocolates (51 per cent sugar), but in bottled salad dressing (30 per cent) and nondairy cream substitutes (65 per cent). Packaged breakfast cereals (as much as 57 per cent sugar) are a major source.

This microscopic cross section of a tooth's crown shows a cavity in the making: Acids produced by bacterial colonies called plaque have eaten through the protective enamel coating at left, leaving the soft underlying tissue open to infection. The microorganisms thrive on sugary foods, particularly sticky forms such as caramel that adhere to the teeth for long periods.

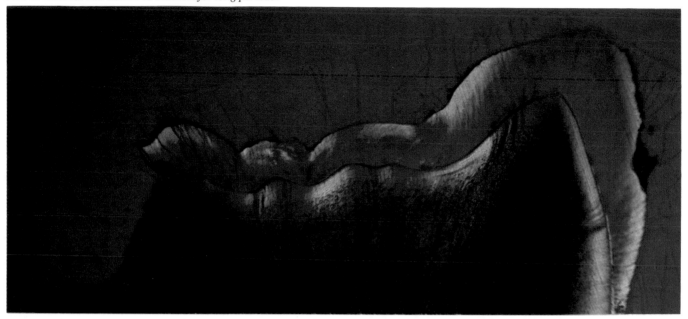

Dentists long believed that sugar caused cavities. Pierre Fauchard, the Frenchman who founded the profession in the 18th Century, wrote that "sugary food contributes not a little to the destruction of teeth." But proof was elusive because a host of additional factors also affect tooth decay: childhood nutrition, the ratio between fat and carbohydrate in the diet, genetic differences and the amount of naturally occurring fluoride minerals in the water, for example.

The first conclusive evidence against sugar emerged from World Wars I and II. During the wars, when sugar was rationed and consumption dropped dramatically, the cavity rate declined as well. In 1914, for example, roughly 90 per cent of German seven-year-olds had cavities; by 1919, after per capita sugar consumption declined from 55 to 30 pounds a year, the cavity figure had dropped to 78 per cent—only to rebound in the ensuing years as sugar consumption resumed at the old rate. Dental studies after World War II revealed similar patterns in Norway, England, Italy, Switzerland, France and Japan. This evidence proved to be accurate but misleading. Soon after World War II, an elaborate five-year Swedish study eliminated all doubt about the role of sugar in tooth decay—and surprised dentists by revealing that the amount of sugar consumed is not particularly important. The amount of tooth decay depends on the type of sugary food and the timing of meals.

In this classic study, 436 residents of a mental hospital in Vipeholm, Sweden, were first fed well-balanced meals containing little sugar four times a day for a year. Then they were divided into groups and fed different types of sugar in addition to the basic diet: One group consumed dissolved sugar daily with meals, one ate a sugary bread with meals, and others ate various amounts of chocolate, caramel or toffee between meals. (This invaluable study could not be repeated today. Experiments on subjects whose participation may not be truly voluntary, such as mental patients and prison inmates, are proscribed by modern ethical standards, along with human experiments that risk permanent injury.)

The sugar solution that accompanied meals caused only a slight increase in cavities, regardless of the amount of sugar consumed—some subjects were given 10 ounces per day. The sweet bread, which contained only one sixth as much sugar as the solution, caused roughly the same increase. But candies that were eaten between meals caused a dramatic increase in cavities. The practical implications were obvious: Between-meal sweets were the primary cause of cavities.

The cause—and prevention—of cavities

Following the Vipeholm experiments, other research on both laboratory rats and humans revealed how cavities occur—and how they can be prevented. Bacteria were long known to be the direct cause of tooth decay. The mouth is always inhabited by a great variety of microbes, which combine with debris from food and from dead cells to form dental plaque—a sticky, jelly-like film that covers the teeth. Plaque ordinarily is harmless. But when any carbohydrate food—sugar is one type—enters the mouth, chemicals released by the plaque's bacteria quickly ferment the carbohydrate, forming lactic acid, a corrosive that can eat through a tooth's protective layer of enamel to form a cavity.

Healthy teeth—partly the result of good childhood nutrition that has supplied plenty of calcium, phosphorus and vitamins A, C and D—are relatively impervious to attack. In recent years this natural resistance to decay has been enhanced by fluoride compounds, which form a stronger, less porous crystal structure in the tooth enamel. Where drinking water does not naturally contain adequate amounts of fluoride (about one part per million), this compound often is added to the water. Dentists may also recommend that children up to the age of 13 take fluoride supplements and use toothpastes containing fluorides.

In addition, the teeth have an impressive array of active defenders against tooth decay. Among them are enzymes and antibodies that attack the harmful bacteria (a fact that has prompted scientists to dream of curing tooth decay with a vaccine to stimulate production of such bacteria killers). Perhaps the most important defense against decay is provided by saliva, which dilutes and neutralizes the acid; if salivary flow decreases—a side effect of many drugs, including antihistamines and tranquilizers—cavities quickly multiply. Salivary flow also drops precipitously during sleep—the reason that midnight snacks cause cavities and that flossing and brushing the teeth are particularly important at bedtime.

This array of defenses proves virtually impregnable so long as the carbohydrates eaten are the complex type—potatoes, pasta, grains, bread and similar foods. Although such foods can cause cavities, they rarely do; their complex molecules are difficult to ferment, so bacteria in the mouth generate only mild acid. Simple carbohydrates, however, are very readily fermented. Such simple carbohydrates include glucose and fructose, the natural sugars that give sweetness to fruit and honey, and sucrose (the chemical name for table sugar). One of the bacteria in the mouth, *Streptoccocus mutans,* thrives on these readily digestible sugars, producing concentrated lactic acid that eats through weak spots in tooth enamel. When this shield is breached, a cavity develops and becomes a harbor for bacteria and the food debris they ferment. Unless a dentist cleans and fills the cavity to block further erosion by acid, the tooth eventually will rot away.

The best way to prevent tooth decay is to control the amount of acid fermented by oral bacteria. As the Vipeholm study proved, it is crucial to limit the frequency of sugary snacks. Any consumption of sugars bathes the teeth with acid for about 30 minutes; after this microscopic assault the enamel needs three hours to rebuild to its previous strength. Thus the less often the teeth are exposed to attack from sugars, the less decay. Occasional binges on sweets cause less harm because they permit tooth enamel time to recover. And sweets eaten with meals also are less damaging—bacteria in the mouth produce acid then anyway.

Although between-meal snacks can be a boon to overall health—they assure a steady absorption of nutrients, help control weight and minimize strain on the digestive system—they are the chief villains in tooth decay. The modern epidemic of cavities can be largely blamed on between-meal snacks—which are principally sweets. Early in the century, such eating on the run was virtually unknown; today it accounts for about 15 per cent of the average daily calorie consumption in the United States.

The type of snack also is critical. The Vipeholm study showed that sugary foods retained in the mouth are particularly harmful, because saliva dissolves them quite slowly. Sweet liquids, such as fruit juices and soft drinks, cause few cavities because they are washed away in a minute or less; ice cream remains for about two minutes. Foods such as caramel, honey, chocolate and cookies, however, adhere to teeth and mouth tissues for at least five minutes. Bread with honey and butter remains for seven and a half minutes because the starch in bread renders sugar particularly sticky—the same reason that cookies, cakes and pastries are so damaging. Worst of all are candies that dissolve slowly if at all, such as jelly beans, suckers, lozenges and chewing gum.

The implications are clear. If you must eat sweets between meals, try to forego hard-to-dissolve foods: chocolate, caramel, toffee, raisins, dates, figs, and all sweet starchy foods, such as doughnuts, cookies, and bread with jam. Instead, choose soft drinks, ice cream, fresh fruits or nuts.

The final consideration in preventing cavities is the concentration of sugar in food. The sugar in candy is so concentrated that it penetrates the dental plaque long before saliva can wash it away. Certain foods such as bananas, oranges, soft drinks and fruit juices have a larger total amount of sugar, but rarely cause cavities because the sugar concentration is low. Abraham E. Nizel, professor of dentistry at Tufts University, offers this example: Although an apple contains more sugar than an ounce of presweetened breakfast cereal, it has less effect on the teeth because the cereal is more than 50 per cent sucrose while the apple's water content brings its sugar concentration to only about 10 per cent.

Why milk makes some people sick

Second only to tooth decay as a diet-caused disease is the digestive upset produced by milk. As many as 70 per cent of the people in the world are born with an inherited inability to digest lactose—a sugar that is the primary carbohydrate in dairy products and makes up about 5 per cent of cow's milk. The incidence of this trait varies widely by ethnic group, however: Only 5 per cent of the white population in Western Europe cannot digest milk—presumably because their ancestors depended on dairy cattle for survival; about 15 per cent of white Americans are affected. But according to some estimates as many as seven out of 10 among black Americans, Mexicans, Jews and Mediterranean peoples such as Arabs and Greeks, and nine out of 10 Orientals and Africans cannot digest lactose.

Such statistics are difficult to verify; some people apparently feel sick after drinking milk because they think they will. Even allowing for psychosomatic effects, though, lactose intolerance remains an important problem. Although not dangerous, it makes its victims feel very sick. It is the leading cause of chronic abdominal pain among adolescents. A study of 80 children who were treated for recurring abdominal pain at Children's Hospital in Boston revealed that 40 per cent of the complaints were due to lactose intolerance; among black and Mexican-American children, the rate was 75 per cent.

The ill effects of milk were not fully appreciated until a humanitarian effort by dairy-rich countries of the West backfired. Shipments of milk powder were sent as gifts to many parts of the world where undernourishment was endemic— but where the inhabitants had inherited lactose intolerance. Colombian Indians refused to drink reconstituted milk and used it instead to paint their huts. Navajo Indians discarded government-issued milk rather than suffer diarrhea, and some African tribes threw away gifts of milk, complaining that it harbored evil spirits.

Underlying this political and medical brouhaha is an inherited shortage of the intestinal enzyme lactase, needed to digest lactose. Virtually all babies possess adequate amounts of this enzyme—otherwise they could not digest their mothers' milk—but in many individuals lactase levels fall during the years after weaning. Gradually the ability to digest milk declines, although it seldom entirely disappears; most lactose-intolerant people can drink a single glass without ill effects.

Most sufferers quickly learn to avoid milk. But in doing so they may deprive themselves of needed nutrients. Studies at the Mayo Clinic in Rochester, Minnesota, implicated lactose intolerance in osteoporosis, a common disease of the elderly (particularly women), in which the bones shrink and become brittle because of a lack of calcium—richly provided by milk. Of 30 patients suffering from osteoporosis, more than 25 per cent were lactose intolerant.

To get enough of milk's valuable ingredients, anyone who is hypersensitive to milk should try alternatives before forsaking dairy products. Many people can tolerate small amounts of milk with meals, particularly if the milk is not ice-cold—cold milk moves through their intestines too rapidly for lactose absorption. Others can use dairy products that contain less lactose, such as hard cheese, yogurt and buttermilk; an ounce of cheddar cheese, for example, contains about as much calcium as a cup of milk, but less than a tenth of the lactose. And the offending lactose can be neutralized in ordinary milk by adding the enzyme lactase (available at pharmacies), which breaks lactose down into two simple, readily digestible sugars, galactose and glucose.

Food allergy: facts and fictions

Milk also is one of the foods commonly implicated in food allergy, a separate type of food-caused ailment. Many so-called allergies are psychological reactions to foods rather than the physical reactions of true allergies—as researchers at the National Jewish Hospital in Denver demonstrated. In tests there on children, laboratory assistants filled capsules with suspected allergy-causing foods. Then a doctor—one who was ignorant of the contents—watched each patient swallow the capsules and observed the reaction. If the reaction was ambiguous the test was repeated, sometimes with capsules containing nothing but sugar. Of 81 patients tested, only one third reacted to the suspected foods; two thirds apparently suffered from psychosomatic reactions. Such reactions are real and troublesome, but they are not allergies.

For reasons not fully understood, infants and children younger than three are especially prone to food allergies. Most of these conditions disappear by adolescence, never to return. Adults with a history of other allergies are particularly susceptible to food allergies; in such cases the food allergy often occurs only during attacks of the other allergy.

Although it is possible to become allergic to virtually any food, a handful of staples elicits nearly all of the proven allergies. Nuts set off almost half the reactions, eggs (usually the whites) and milk about a fifth; most of the remainder are caused by shellfish, flour, soybean products and the commonly used—and generally safe—food dye, Yellow No. 5. Most foods traditionally blamed for allergies, such as fish,

chocolate, cola drinks and tomatoes, rarely cause true allergies; reactions to them appear to be mainly psychosomatic.

The basic mechanism of all true food allergies is the same: Antibodies, the microscopic sentinels that protect the body from invaders by attacking and removing them, are accidentally programed to attack certain food proteins as well. This action usually occurs in the gastrointestinal tract, causing vomiting, abdominal pain and diarrhea. If the proteins filter unhindered through the intestinal wall into the blood and lymph systems, dispersing throughout the body, antibodies in the skin may generate hives, rashes, swelling and itching; antibodies in the lungs may cause asthma and a stuffy nose. A handful of food allergy victims may experience an immediate, potentially deadly reaction called anaphylactic shock: respiratory distress, vomiting, cramps and diarrhea. Within 15 minutes the victim can collapse and die.

Because drugs do not cure food allergies, there is only one solution: Avoid the offending food, a task that requires constant vigilance because the most common villains are staples of Western cuisine. Sufferers must scrutinize the labels on all prepared foods (particularly for Yellow No. 5) and question waiters and chefs when dining out. In addition, some allergy victims have to find alternate sources of essential nutrients, such as the calcium and protein in milk.

If food is unquestionably a cause of allergies and tooth decay, its role in such scourges as heart attack, stroke and cancer remains controversial. Yet enough is known to influence the choice of what to eat. A handful of foods almost certainly bring on these three deadly ailments, and at least one type of food may help prevent cancer.

Both heart attacks and strokes have now been traced to the consumption of large amounts of salty food. The salt contributes to high blood pressure—hypertension—which precipitates many strokes. Hypertension also increases the risk of heart attack; a blood pressure reading of 170/95 (about 130/70 is considered normal) increases the chance of heart attack fourfold.

Scientists first speculated in 1904 that salt contributed to hypertension, and have been amassing evidence ever since, comparing peoples who traditionally eat a great deal of salt with those who do not: bushmen of the Kalahari Desert, Congo pygmies, Greenland Eskimos, Cook Islanders and the Yanomamo Indians of Brazil among others. Without exception, the studies showed that hypertension is a problem only where salty foods are common. The research singles out salt as the primary villain, outweighing such frequently cited factors as stress, crowding, a sedentary lifestyle or obesity. A 1976 study of the Qash'qai nomads of Iran, primitive sheep-herders who are active and lean but addicted to salty foods, revealed that roughly 15 per cent of the adults had hypertension. And when a Harvard University team investigated several tribes on the Solomon Islands, the scientists found that Lau fishermen, who boil their food in sea water, had a much higher hypertension rate than neighboring tribes who lived similar lives but cooked with fresh water.

Salt contributes to hypertension because it is a compound containing the element sodium, which serves to regulate the passage of fluids through the walls of tissue cells. The body needs about .007 ounce of sodium daily for this purpose, the amount in about $^1/_{10}$ teaspoon of salt; in industrialized nations, however, the average person's daily consumption is 10 to 40 times this amount. The excess sodium can gradually alter the transmission of fluids into and out of cells so that tissues expand slightly, squeezing blood vessels and raising blood pressure. In industrialized nations blood pressure ascends steadily during adulthood, and three people out of four develop hypertension by the time they reach age 60; in other regions, where little salt is consumed, blood pressure is unchanged throughout adulthood.

Drugs can control hypertension, but a better cure and the only preventive is reduced consumption of sodium. One fourth of the average intake cannot be effectively regulated, because the mineral occurs naturally in raw foods. But the remainder is avoidable because it comes from salt—one third of it added during cooking and at the table, nearly two thirds added during industrial food processing.

Cutting salt intake—one and a half teaspoons per day is the recommended maximum—is simple so long as home-made foods are eaten: Reduce the amount of salt used in recipes, forego salty seasonings such as soy sauce and refrain

from adding salt at the table. But industrially processed foods are the primary source of sodium. Commercially frozen peas have 100 times as much sodium as fresh peas, and canned peas contain more than 200 times as much; use of such foods must be restricted if the consumption of sodium is to be held within recommended limits.

More complicated than the case implicating salt in heart attacks and stroke is the one against a particular group of foods, those that contain certain types of fats. These fats are linked to clogging of the arteries by fatty deposits—the condition called atherosclerosis—that can bring on a stroke if the clogging is in a brain artery, a heart attack if in a heart artery. The plugs that clog the arteries are composed mostly of a fatty compound called cholesterol, and many heart at-

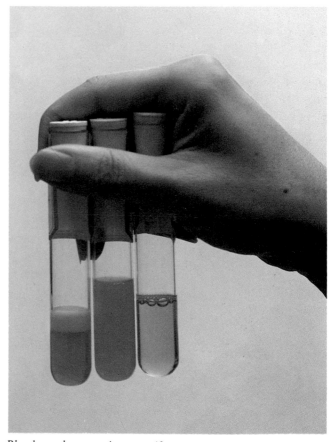

Blood samples, spun in a centrifuge to separate components, provide a quick visual check of fats that may cause heart ailments. The waxy residue at left is fat unprocessed because of a liver defect. The cloudy middle sample suggests an excess of fats called triglycerides. The clear plasma is inconclusive—it could contain excess cholesterol, detectable only by further analysis.

tack victims have high levels of cholesterol in their blood.

At first researchers blamed atherosclerosis on the amount of cholesterol in the diet—primarily from egg yolks, which contain about 40 per cent of the total cholesterol consumed in most Western countries, but also from dairy products, red meat and shellfish. This turned out to be an oversimplification. More than half the body's cholesterol is manufactured by the liver rather than ingested, and the amount manufactured depends more on the types of fat eaten than on the consumption of cholesterol itself. Saturated fats—the type that predominates in meat, eggs and dairy products—dramatically increase cholesterol in the blood; monounsaturated fats, found in peanut oil and olive oil, have no effect; and polyunsaturated fats, which predominate in fruits, vegetables and other plant foods, tend to reduce cholesterol levels.

The more saturated fats eaten, the higher the level of cholesterol—and the greater the risk of heart attack or stroke. In the United States, for example, a middle-aged man whose cholesterol level ranks in the top 20 per cent is twice as likely to have a heart attack as a man with a level in the bottom 40 per cent.

Although some experts dispute the role of fats in disease, the statistical evidence led public health authorities in many countries to launch unprecedented campaigns to change diets by reducing fats to about 30 per cent of total calorie consumption—a 9 per cent reduction—and to cut saturated fats to about 10 per cent of total calories. These recommendations require drastic alterations in customary menus: roughly half as many eggs; one fifth less meat, fish and poultry; and one sixth less fat and oil. In addition, consumption of grain products, fruits, vegetables and skim milk would have to increase in order to supply calories and nutrients previously provided by animal fats.

The diet resulting from such changes is not so much an innovation as a throwback to traditional types of fare that until the 19th Century were standard everywhere and still predominate in China, southern Italy, Greece, the Middle East and many other regions that have little heart disease. The campaign seems to be producing the desired effect. In the United States, for example, consumption of fatty foods decreased between 1950 and 1974: that of eggs dropped 26 per cent, milk and cream 31 per cent, butter 64 per cent and lard 77 per cent.

The elusive cancer connection

Unlike the broad consensus blaming animal fats for circulatory ailments, scientific opinion about the link between foods and cancer abounds with conflicting theories, a reflection of cancer's complexity. The modern diet contains hundreds of foods and more than 40 distinct nutrients, all constantly changing and interacting during cooking and digestion to form thousands of organic compounds. Any one of these can play a part in cancer. Many scientists—among them Dr. Ernst Wynder of the American Health Foundation, who demonstrated that cigarettes cause cancer—maintain that nearly half of all cancer cases in the United States arise from diet.

Some connections between cancer and diet are fairly firmly established. Obesity is one. Fat women have a greater risk of cancer of the uterus. Women who are not necessarily obese but eat a high-fat diet have an increased risk of breast cancer and men on such a diet have a heightened risk of prostate cancer. In addition, some substances found in food—naturally occurring compounds, not synthetic additives introduced by modern processing—cause cancer.

The most potent of these natural carcinogens are the aflatoxins, produced by molds that often infest foods. The hazards of aflatoxins in peanuts were first discovered in Africa (pages 102-103); but the hardy molds also grow on a variety of Western foodstuffs, including other nuts as well as corn, wheat, rice, milk and perhaps even cheese. Close inspection by government agencies keeps aflatoxin-contaminated produce from being sold, but the mold can develop after the food is taken home. Moldy bread, for example, can harbor aflatoxin. The poison is not inactivated by cooking or refrigeration, so moldy parts of any food should be pared away.

A more serious source of cancer in industrialized countries is alcohol. Not only does it interact with tobacco to increase the risk of cancer among smokers, but it can also cause cancers of the mouth, larynx, esophagus and liver. Even small amounts—less than two ounces of whiskey or two

In Finland, a war on fatty foods

The Finnish province of North Karelia, hard by the Soviet border, is plagued by one of the world's highest death rates from heart disease. Not coincidentally, the North Karelians, like most Finns, consume a diet unusually high in saturated fats—believed to increase the risk of circulatory ailments. So in 1972 the Finnish government set up a program to help the North Karelians alter their diets and living habits.

The government sent doctors, nurses and technicians to conduct classes and visit households and businesses, informing people of the dangers of smoking, high blood pressure and a high-fat diet. Leaflets, posters and radio announcements pressed the message. Medical monitoring stations were set up to collect data and help the North Karelians keep track of their health. The campaign was a success: By 1977, the incidence of heart attacks among middle-aged men in North Karelia had declined 16 per cent, that of strokes 38 per cent.

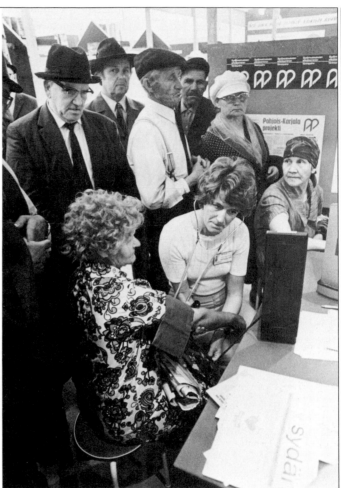

At the Karelian Fair in 1973, a woman has her blood pressure measured as part of a campaign to help Finns monitor their progress in altering diet to combat heart disease.

Questioning a lumberjack, a Finnish doctor (right) researches the loggers' diet—once so rich it had astounded American experts visiting in 1956. One observer watched loggers take thick slabs of cheese, "smear them a quarter of an inch deep with butter and eat them, with a beer, as an after-sauna snack."

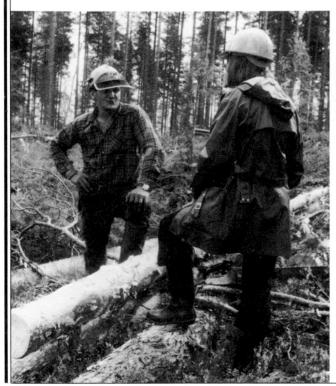

beers per day—increase the risk of cancer, but most authorities believe that this danger is more than offset by the established benefit of moderate drinking in preventing heart attacks. However, heavy drinkers—who already risk heart disease, hypertension and cirrhosis of the liver—face the same cancer risk as two-pack-a-day smokers. A study of cancer patients in East Orange, New Jersey, found that those who drank from one to six ounces of whiskey per day (or equivalent amounts of beer or wine) had three times the cancer risk of teetotalers. Those who drank between six and nine drinks per day had 15 times the nondrinkers' risk.

But the most important connection between diet and cancer may be a link between fatty foods and cancer of the colon, responsible for 50,000 deaths annually in the United States. Americans get about 40 per cent of their daily calories from fat, compared to about 15 per cent in Japan; the Japanese rate for colon cancer is less than one fourth that in the United States. Similarly low rates of colon cancer have been observed in other countries where fat consumption is low, including Costa Rica, Bulgaria and Rhodesia.

Further evidence implicating fat—any kind, saturated or not—comes from laboratory experiments and knowledge of the fat-digestion process. When two groups of rats eat equal amounts of a cancer-causing chemical, the rats on a fatty diet develop nearly twice as many tumors as those on a low-fat diet. The effect, in humans as well, is believed to be related to the actions of bile acids, produced by the liver and secreted into the intestine, where the fats are emulsified and digested; the more fat eaten, the more bile acids are present. The acids may promote colon cancer. Eating much fat may also alter the mixture of intestinal bacteria, favoring those types that break down bile acids into tumor-promoting compounds.

Methods of food preparation likewise play a part in cancer because they change the food's chemical make-up and may introduce cancer-causing compounds. Japan's stomach cancer rate—48 times the rate anywhere else—is blamed largely on broiled and salty foods. An average Japanese uses about 35 pounds of salt per year, four times as much as most Americans and Europeans. Dried fish, a staple of Japanese cuisine, contains as much as 20 per cent salt and is generally, said

A cancer cause in moldy peanuts

From thatched peanut-storage huts in Africa (opposite) to corncribs in Canada lurks a natural troublemaker named *Aspergillus flavus*. A fungus that thrives in moist environments on nuts, beans, corn and other grains, it produces a poison, aflatoxin, that causes cancer.

The danger of aflatoxin has been known since the 1960s, when a rash of turkey deaths in England was traced to feed tainted by the mold. Soon researchers studying cancer in humans indicted aflatoxin: People in regions where aflatoxin contamination was worst—Southeast Asia and tropical Africa—had among the highest liver cancer rates in the world.

Most governments have since started monitoring susceptible crops and urging growers and users to store such foods in dry, well-ventilated places. But even nations with strict controls and advanced food-storage practices are not free of the problem: Corn contaminated by aflatoxin was discovered in the United States and banned from sale in 1977.

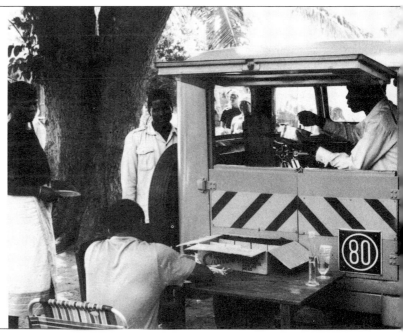

In a study of the fungus poison aflatoxin, a woman in Mozambique —where the incidence of liver cancer, linked to aflatoxin, is the world's highest—delivers a sample of a meal to a mobile health unit for later analysis. The research pinpointed one source of aflatoxin in a breakfast staple, boiled peanuts—its soggy leftovers provided an ideal culture for the mold.

Toshio Oiso of the National Institute for Nutrition, "broiled until it is burned black." Laboratory experiments indicate that salt and high-temperature cooking—sautéing, browning and charcoal-broiling—create chemicals like those that cause cancer. Presumably such hazards also accompany the broiled and fried foods favored in the West.

The virtues of fiber

In contrast to the dangers posed by many foods are the benefits attributed to one component of food: fiber, which is not a nutritional foodstuff but is indigestible roughage. It is held to prevent cancer of the colon and is a well-established treatment for a number of less serious intestinal disorders.

The checkered history of fiber in nutrition, a classic illustration of the changeability of dietary advice, commenced in pre-Christian times; Hippocrates urged patients to eat abundantly of vegetables, fruit and wheatmeal bread "for the salutory effects upon the bowels." Most authorities echoed this advice through the 19th Century. In the 1830s Sylvester Graham—an evangelist for Christianity and vegetarianism,

remembered today in graham crackers and graham flour—grew wealthy by preaching that ill health was the product of too rich a diet, and that the right food would save not only lives but immortal souls. To a Victorian audience obsessed with dyspepsia and constipation, Graham touted the virtues of bran, the outer husk of the wheat kernel, usually removed from white flour. "Every farmer knows that if his horse has straw cut with his grain, he does well enough. Just so it is with the human species. Man needs bran in his bread," Graham thundered from his pulpit. He also maintained that chicken pie caused cholera (as did lewdness), condiments caused insanity and meat led to sexual excesses.

Forty years later a Seventh-day Adventist physician, Dr. John Harvey Kellogg—founder of the Kellogg breakfast-cereal empire—took up the bran crusade. Dr. Kellogg, who supervised a posh sanatorium in Battle Creek, Michigan, treated and counseled millionaires—Henry Ford, John D. Rockefeller and Harvey Firestone, among others. Dr. Kellogg believed that disease was caused by poisoned intestines, and he prescribed several treatments: a daily enema; a purify-

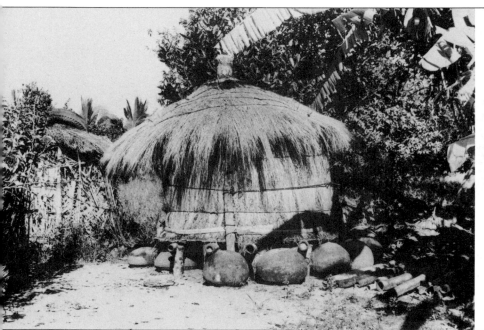

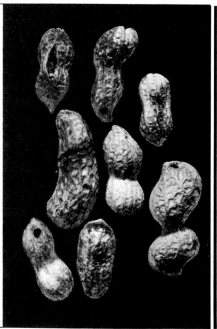

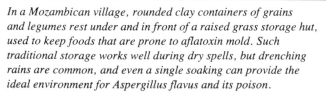

In a Mozambican village, rounded clay containers of grains and legumes rest under and in front of a raised grass storage hut, used to keep foods that are prone to aflatoxin mold. Such traditional storage works well during dry spells, but drenching rains are common, and even a single soaking can provide the ideal environment for Aspergillus flavus and its poison.

Holes, pits and scars in the shells of the Mozambican peanuts above suggest that these nuts are contaminated by aflatoxin. Termites bore into the shells, admitting fungus spores that find a moist, hospitable place to grow and release aflatoxin.

ing meat-free regimen he called nature's broom, made up of lettuce, celery, cucumbers, green corn, cabbage and turnips; and in addition, quantities of bran, stale graham bread and breakfast cereals. By the 1890s his cereals were marketed nationwide; a great commercial battle between Dr. Kellogg and one of his imitators, Charles W. Post, ensued, turning Battle Creek into a boom town—and spreading the gospel of fiber around the world.

But in the early 20th Century fiber fell into disfavor. Roughage was considered an irritant and blamed for ulcers, dyspepsia and the irritable-bowel syndrome—chronic bloating, cramps and alternating diarrhea and constipation. As late as the 1960s, doctors prescribed bland, fiber-free diets for patients with gastrointestinal problems.

Then in the early 1970s Denis Burkitt—a British surgeon already famous for research into the cancer that bears his name, Burkitt's lymphoma—began a fiber crusade that earned him the sobriquet, "the Bran Man." Citing the low colon cancer rate among Africans who eat much fiber and the high rate among Europeans who do not, Burkitt argued that fiber prevents the cancer. Many physicians rushed to act on Burkitt's admittedly preliminary observations, and roughage returned to general favor, this time as both a cancer preventive and a cure for gastrointestinal ills.

The name now given roughage is somewhat misleading. Fiber is not fibrous; celery, for example, which looks and feels fibrous, has less fiber than seemingly fiber-free baking chocolate (chart, pages 161-171). Furthermore, fiber is no single substance but a potpourri of chemicals from the walls of plant cells; the mixture varies from plant to plant. Even the measurement of fiber is deceptive. What is generally listed as "fiber" in labels and advertisements is crude fiber, the residue left after the food is dissolved in chemicals. This analytic process bears little resemblance to human digestion and underestimates the true amount of fiber in food, called dietary fiber, by as much as 50 per cent.

By any name, fiber seems to help. Laboratory experiments indicate it absorbs bile acids and carcinogens, thus protecting the colon; it also may absorb cholesterol and thus help prevent heart attacks. Fiber also tips the balance of bacteria in the colon toward those bacteria that do not convert bile acids into tumor-producing compounds. Even the cautious National Cancer Institute stated, "A generous intake of dietary fiber would seem prudent."

Fiber is available in fresh fruits, vegetables and unrefined grains. A bowl of all-bran cereal or several slices of whole-grain bread supply the daily requirement. Fiber is a two-edged sword, however. It should be added to the diet gradually; otherwise, abdominal cramps and gas may appear until the digestive tract can adjust. And very large quantities of fiber can do harm; they may hinder the absorption of vita-

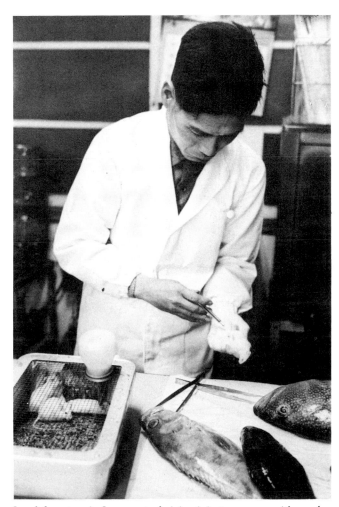

In a laboratory in Japan, a technician injects a mouse with a pulp made from salted fish like those on the table, in an attempt to induce stomach cancer. The experiment has special significance for the Japanese: It may show a link between their stomach-cancer rate—the world's highest—and their national diet, which includes large amounts of heavily salted foods.

mins and minerals or cause a dangerous kink in the intestine.

Although fiber has been most publicized as a colon cancer preventive, it also is a proved treatment for several other intestinal disorders. It draws extra water into the stool, softening it and speeding elimination in constipated people but slowing it in those plagued by diarrhea. The softer stool also eases rectal inflammation, such as hemorrhoids. Fiber can help to cure the irritable-bowel syndrome, often caused by psychological stress that reduces the diameter of the colon, increasing pressure and triggering spastic muscular contractions. Because fiber adds bulk to the stool, it increases the colon diameter and prevents muscle spasms.

Fiber is now recommended to prevent the dangerous intestinal disease called diverticulosis—a remarkable reversal in medical opinion, which as recently as the 1960s blamed fiber itself for this disorder. As a low-fiber diet narrows the colon, the heightened pressure inside tends to push the intestinal lining through weak points in the surrounding muscle wall. The resulting pockets, called diverticula, trap fragments of stool, become inflamed and eventually bleed or rupture, sometimes infecting the entire abdominal cavity. Modern medical textbooks universally—if abashedly—recommend a high-fiber diet for both prevention and treatment; one notes that ''contrary to prior opinion, a bland diet is *not* indicated for persons with diverticulosis.''

Coping with diabetes

The one disorder that transcends the normal categories of dietary diseases is diabetes. It is not, as was long believed, brought on by eating too much sugar. Yet diet plays a part in both its cause and its treatment.

Diabetes is a failure of the body's energy-regulating system and affects every part of the body. Despite strides during the 20th Century in treating the disease with drugs, it remains the No. 3 killer. The exact death toll is impossible to determine—death certificates usually blame complications rather than diabetes itself—but Dr. Howard S. Traisman of the Northwestern University Medical School estimates that it causes 300,000 deaths annually in the United States alone.

Diabetes was blamed on sugar because its victims cannot process glucose, the special form of sugar that provides most energy. The digestive system transforms foods into glucose, which is absorbed into cells and converted into energy at the command of a chemical middleman, the hormone insulin, produced by the pancreas gland. This system can go awry if either the pancreas fails to secrete insulin or the energy-generating cells fail to react to the hormone. The body, unable to tap the plentiful supplies of glucose, gets its energy by consuming its reserves of fats and proteins. Unless careful treatment is provided, the result is blindness, kidney failure, heart failure or a rapid wasting away to death.

Failure of the pancreas, which generally strikes children between the ages of 10 and 12, is the more serious cause of the disease. The complex causes of so-called juvenile diabetes have emerged only recently. Researchers long believed that several genetic flaws, rather than any single one, were implicated in diabetes. But this explains only part of the problem. Studies of identical twins revealed that when one child develops juvenile diabetes, there is only a 50-50 chance that the other twin also will get the disease; if diabetes were caused solely by genes, the correspondence would be 100 per cent. Scientists now are finding evidence that several childhood viruses, among them German measles, shingles and mumps, can destroy pancreatic cells of susceptible people, perhaps because of some inherited fault. A conjunction of these two factors—virus exposure and genetic defect—may be the actual cause of juvenile diabetes.

The onset of juvenile diabetes is quite sudden, usually a matter of days. The symptoms are frequent urination, as the kidneys attempt to eliminate excess glucose; constant thirst, an attempt to replenish the lost water supply; rapid weight loss, as the body burns fats and proteins in place of glucose; weakness and fatigue; and a constant craving for food. Untreated, a juvenile diabetic soon falls into a coma and dies. Prior to the 20th Century the end could be staved off for about two years with a 400-calorie diet that excluded all sources of glucose, but such measures added starvation to the ravages of diabetes and merely postponed the inevitable.

This was the grim prospect in 1921, when Dr. Frederick Banting, a 30-year-old surgeon, and Charles Best, a 22-year-

An automatic pump to control blood sugar

Looking like a small transistor radio and weighing less than a pound, the battery-operated device pictured at near right may revolutionize the care of diabetics. Called a portable infusion pump, it is in effect an external replacement for the pancreas, the sugar-regulating organ whose failure is the cause of diabetes.

Worn on a belt 24 hours a day, the pump trickles insulin at a slow and steady rate through a needle into the tissue of a diabetic's abdomen. It thus maintains normal blood-sugar levels in much the same way that a healthy pancreas does. To compensate for the normal rise in blood sugar that follows eating, a diabetic can increase the insulin dosage; he merely switches the pump from its automatic, slow-drip setting to a manual one and gives himself more of the vital hormone.

The portable infusion pump, introduced by researchers at Case Western Reserve University in the 1970s and approved for general use in 1976, was designed initially to administer drugs to cancer patients. Because the pump delivers a steady flow of insulin and thereby reduces fluctuations in the amounts of sugar in the blood, doctors believe it may help eliminate some of the disease's long-term complications—including blindness, kidney failure and circulatory problems. To victims of diabetes, however, the pump brings one immediate and overwhelming boon: Because it is worn around the clock, it does away with the daily ritual of injecting insulin.

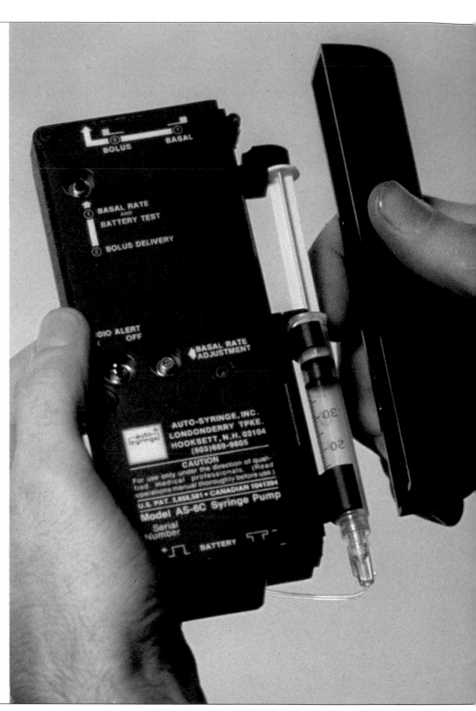

The portable infusion pump holds a one-day supply of insulin in its plastic syringe. The pump runs on a rechargeable battery and has alarms to warn the wearer if the battery is running low or if the insulin is being released improperly. Switches at the top enable the user to administer insulin either automatically (on the setting marked "basal") or manually (on the "bolus" setting).

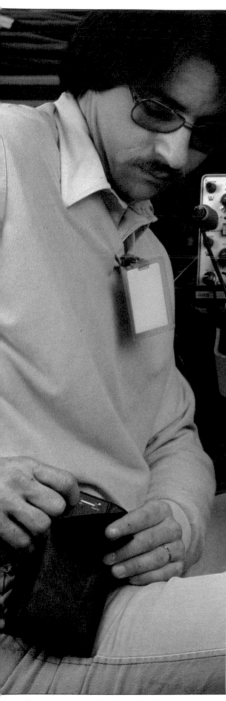

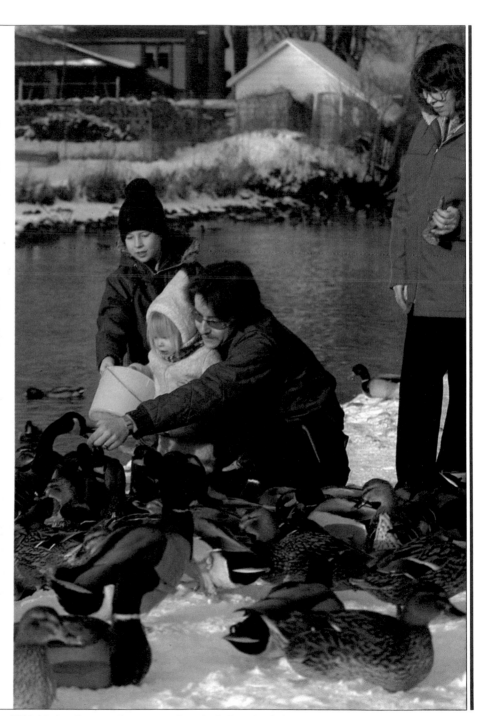

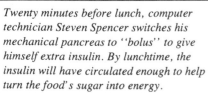

Twenty minutes before lunch, computer technician Steven Spencer switches his mechanical pancreas to ''bolus'' to give himself extra insulin. By lunchtime, the insulin will have circulated enough to help turn the food's sugar into energy.

With his insulin pump hanging unobtrusively from his belt, Spencer helps his children feed a flock of ducks while his wife looks on. Before he began to wear the pump, he would have had to be home at this time of day—5:30 p.m.—giving himself the second of two daily insulin injections. With the pump, however, Spencer need not interrupt his other activities.

old medical student, began research on diabetes at the University of Toronto. They removed a dog's pancreas and injected an extract from it into a diabetic dog; within minutes, the dog's glucose level returned to normal. When they tried the extract on a 14-year-old boy dying of diabetes, the initial response was almost imperceptible, but with subsequent injections the youth improved dramatically; he eventually resumed a normal life.

The extract obtained by Dr. Banting and Best was the hormone insulin. Those with juvenile diabetes must use it daily over a lifetime in conjunction with exercise and a rigid diet *(pages 110-117)*. Refined sugar is forbidden, because it enters the bloodstream so suddenly that injected insulin cannot adequately counteract it. Until recently, diabetic diets limited other carbohydrate foods as well, relying instead on fat and protein for energy. But it is now known that high-carbohydrate diets improve the control of diabetes and help prevent heart disease and other common complications. Such treatment enabled millions with juvenile diabetes—among them television star Mary Tyler Moore, and baseball players Jackie Robinson and Catfish Hunter—to live normal, relatively worry-free lives.

Only about 10 per cent of all diabetics have the juvenile type requiring insulin injections. The others produce their own insulin, but it is ineffective. This "adult-onset" diabetes most often hits the middle-aged and elderly, particularly if they are obese. For centuries scientists blamed excessive sugar consumption. Indeed, as a nation's sugar consumption increased, so did its diabetes rate.

It turns out that there is no difference between the sugar consumption of diabetics and nondiabetics. The Pima Indians of the American Southwest *(page 108)* consume only 50 pounds of sugar per person per year, compared to about 90 for most Americans, yet half the Pima adults have diabetes. On the other hand, sugar-cane cutters in South Africa, nibbling as they work, consume nearly a pound of sugar per day, yet their diabetes rates are low.

Today most scientists believe that heredity and obesity together cause adult-onset diabetes. The adage among diabetes specialists is that "heredity loads the gun but obesity pulls the trigger." A study of middle-aged men in Oslo, Norway, found that moderately fat men were 10 times as likely to develop diabetes as men of normal weight; very fat men were 30 times as likely to get the disease.

The influence of obesity means that adult diabetes can be prevented by a diet that keeps weight under control. Mice genetically susceptible to diabetes do not develop the disease unless they are overfed. The same effect was observed in human populations: In Europe during World War II, the incidence of diabetes declined dramatically whenever food shortages substantially reduced obesity. Some experts blame obesity alone; Dr. Kelly West of the University of Oklahoma maintained that excess fat by itself "is quite capable of producing diabetes" in the absence of any genetic fault.

Diet is not only the preventive, but the primary treatment for adult diabetes. Losing weight usually restores the body's use of glucose to normal. Patients who get their weight down and keep it down still must continue to exercise and to limit their total calorie intake. Those who cannot lose weight sometimes require drugs that improve insulin absorption.

A hard look at the myths
While researchers go on finding more and more ways that eating right can keep people well, they are also discovering that a number of ills often blamed on diet are actually influenced less than had been thought—or not at all—by food.

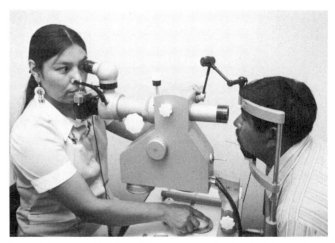

In an Arizona clinic, Pima Indians—a medical technician and a patient—confront each other eyeball to eyeball at a fundus camera, which photographs ruptured blood vessels in the eye, a complication of diabetes. Nearly half the Pima tribe develop the disease; the examination is part of an attempt to learn why.

One of the more startling changes in expert opinion applies to ailments of the digestive system, but also debated are the roles played by diet in arthritis and in the hyperactivity that afflicts many children.

During the first half of the 20th Century, stomach disorders such as acid indigestion and ulcers were treated for months and even years with hourly feedings of milk, toast, cereal, soft-boiled eggs and puréed vegetables—a diet few patients could abide. A clearer understanding of the action of stomach acids, necessary to digestion but sometimes corrosive to the stomach lining, now eases such regimens. Care in eating is still required, however.

Stomach pain, it has been found, can generally be cured by limiting intake of alcohol and caffeine, which stimulate acid secretion; by avoiding spicy foods such as pickles, which irritate the stomach lining; and by avoiding large meals, which tend to stimulate oversecretion of digestive acids. In most cases these measures arrest stomach irritation before a full-fledged ulcer develops. Milk, which was once considered nature's antacid, now is frowned upon; it is emptied rapidly from the stomach and actually stimulates the secretion of acid. If more stringent measures are required, small between-meal snacks of bland foods every two hours are often used, so that food is constantly present to absorb the normal trickle of acid. In extreme cases meat and other high-protein foods are forbidden, because they trigger more acid secretion than do fats and carbohydrates.

For arthritis, another disease traditionally treated with a restrictive diet, the many popular diets are no more effective than copper amulets—with one notable exception: the diet prescribed for gout, an intermittent but excruciating type of arthritis. Gout develops when a surfeit of uric acid, a chemical normally excreted in the urine, forms needle-like crystals in the joints. For centuries gout was blamed on "dissolute and voluptuous Indulgence of Sensual Appetites," to quote one old textbook. Attacks can be triggered by certain foods, but the disease is actually caused by inherited defects that make the body manufacture excess uric acid or fail to eliminate it. Gout usually strikes in middle age, first in the feet, then in other joints; nearly 90 per cent of the victims are men.

Today gout usually is treated with anti-inflammatory drugs, but diet still plays a part in the therapy. Gout patients are advised to avoid peas, beans, sardines, anchovies and organ meats—kidneys, liver, sweetbreads and brains—because these foods trigger the production of large amounts of uric acid. They must avoid heavy drinking bouts, because alcohol interferes with uric acid metabolism and can precipitate an attack. Paradoxically, they must also avoid ascetic fasts or crash diets, because these prevent the kidneys from properly excreting uric acid.

If diet matters less than had been thought in treating ulcers and most forms of arthritis, it seems to have no connection at all to many other ailments for which it has been claimed to be a preventive or sovereign cure. One disorder that attracted much attention in the 1970s was childhood hyperactivity, characterized by agitation, short attention span and learning disabilities. In 1973, California allergist Dr. Benjamin Feingold blamed chemicals called salicylates, which are present in aspirin and also occur naturally in many foods; he also blamed artificial colors and flavors. He based his ideas on well-known adult reactions to aspirin. Many aspirin-intolerant people also react to Yellow No. 5, and Dr. Feingold proposed that other additives also might cause reactions. He prescribed a restrictive, home-cooked diet free of additives and salicylate foods. He claimed that in nearly half of his patients "a favorable response is observed within days after instituting the dietary control."

Experiments, however, failed to find evidence to support the claims made for the Feingold diet. In one study done by J. Ivan Williams of the University of Toronto, 26 hyperactive children on the Feingold diet were fed two types of cookies, one laced with a normal daily dose of artificial colors, the other additive-free. According to observations by parents, teachers and psychologists, the additives did not affect the children's behavior.

Clearly food is neither a preventive nor a cure for every ill afflicting humans. But each year more is learned about the subtle ways it affects health. Enough is now known about the interaction between diet and disease to identify what—and how much—to eat to sustain a vital, active life. ✳

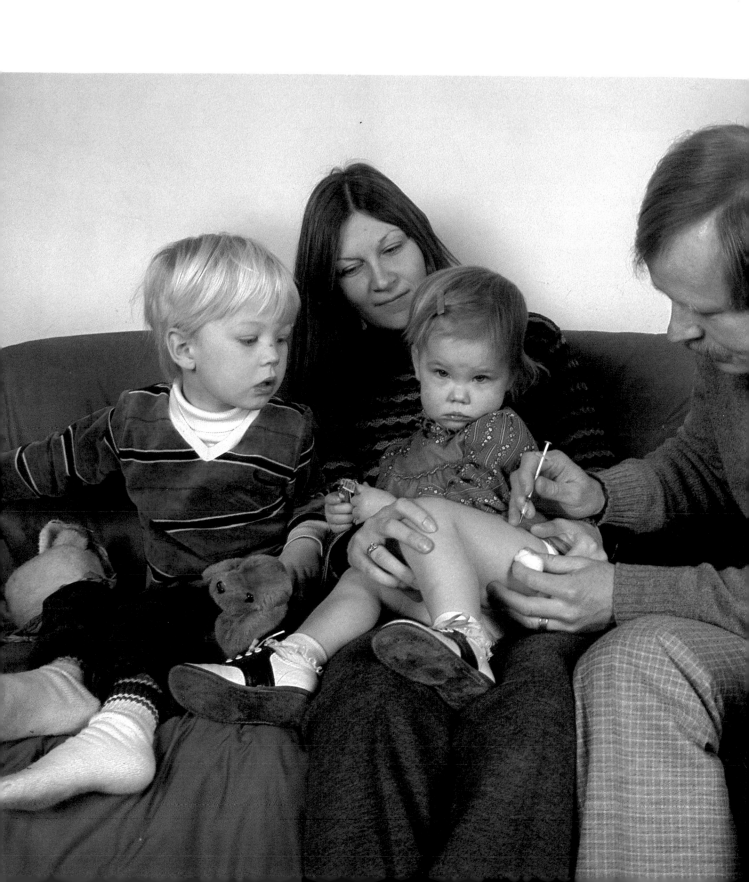

Growing up diabetic

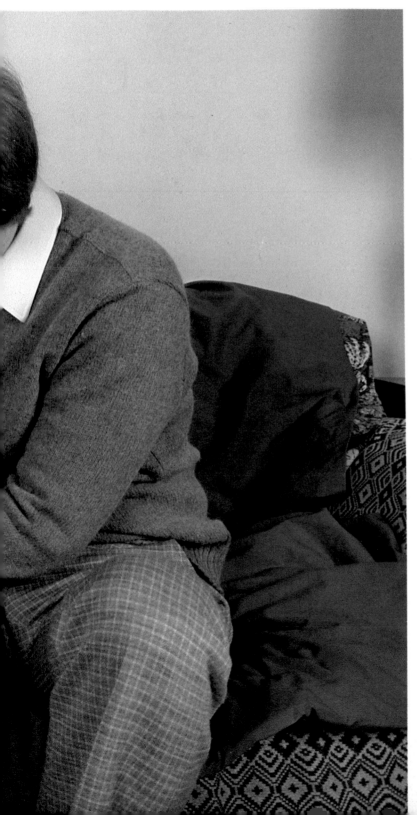

*The morning insulin shot is a family
affair for diabetic Kristin Dahl, who usually
accepts injections uncomplainingly.
She will eventually learn to administer
them herself, making her treatments an
unobtrusive part of normal life.*

"When we first discovered that Jon was diabetic," wrote the parents of a two-year-old Minnesota boy, "the challenge seemed completely overwhelming." Henceforth his diet and exercise would have to be regulated, his condition monitored strictly, and his body supplied with injections of the hormone insulin—all because a crucial organ, the pancreas, suddenly had become unable to produce enough insulin to allow his body to process the sugar glucose, its principal fuel.

But soon after the initial reaction of shock and uncertainty, most children and families confronted by juvenile diabetes learn that almost every young diabetic can, with a few concessions to the disease, enjoy an essentially normal childhood despite his serious and incurable affliction. What is more, most diabetic children today can look forward to a vigorous, rewarding adolescence and adulthood.

By the time they are 12 years old most cope with the disease by themselves. They give themselves insulin shots, usually before breakfast and dinner, and they conduct their own urine or blood tests to monitor the levels of sugar in their blood. They learn how to manage their diets—generally eating foods low in refined sugar, saturated fats and cholesterol, the latter two because diabetics are unusually prone to hardening of the arteries. What is more, they must consume food in amounts and at times designed to correspond with their own activities and the actions of their medications. Snacking becomes a duty. In addition, diabetic children regulate their exercise so that it occurs at approximately the same time—and at the same level of intensity—each day.

These restrictions and requirements somehow get tucked in among the multitude of ordinary things every child does. Young diabetics play actively, participate in athletics, hold down jobs, travel and go out on dinner dates. Thus, although a diabetic child must live in constant awareness of his condition, and must sustain a delicate balance between insulin levels, food intake and exercise, he still, noted the American Diabetes Association, "can take on his share of work around the house, go to a regular school at the usual age and participate in all school activities." Stated one young diabetic: "I control my diabetes. It doesn't control me."

Making treatment an everyday routine

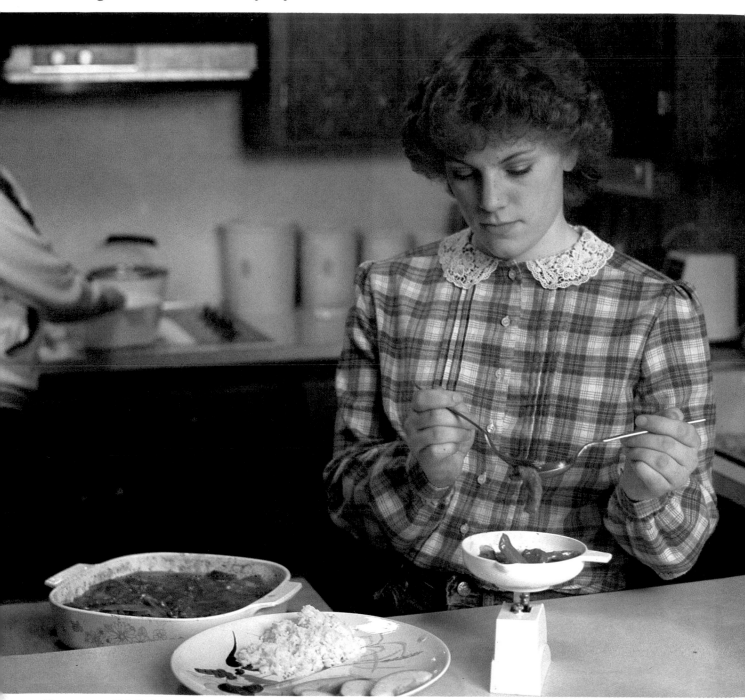

Sixteen-year-old Julie Butler uses a scale to measure exactly three ounces of meat to go with dinnertime portions of rice, apples, Chinese vegetables and milk. Her meal plan, tailored to her age, weight and activity level, must include carefully balanced portions; otherwise, her blood might acquire too much or too little sugar, producing reactions ranging from shakiness to coma.

Eleven-year-old Michael Healey (right) must check the amount
of sugar in his blood three times a day. First, he pricks his
finger with a lancet to draw blood (below), then he places a
drop on a flat, chemically treated strip of plastic (right),
which he inserts into the device on the sink, called a dextrometer.
Its digital dial then registers his blood-sugar level.

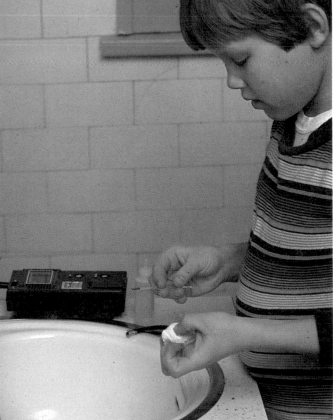

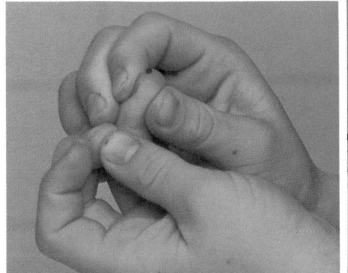

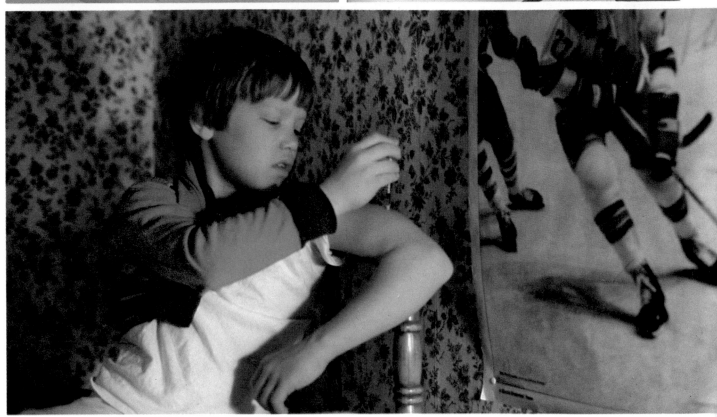

His shirt sleeve rolled up, and his elbow propped for leverage
against the headboard of his bed, Michael gives himself
an insulin injection. This is his morning shot; before dinner he
will administer another. To keep from damaging skin and
tissue, Michael shifts the sites of the injections every few days
among various places on his arms and legs.

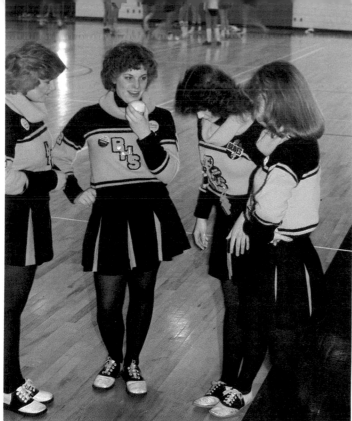

Before cheerleading practice, Julie munches an apple. Because she expends so much energy cheerleading, she needs extra food to keep from depleting her blood sugar and precipitating a so-called insulin reaction, marked by such symptoms as sudden hunger, dizziness, nervousness and pale or moist skin.

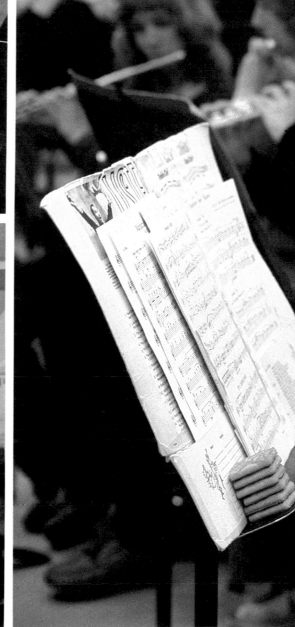

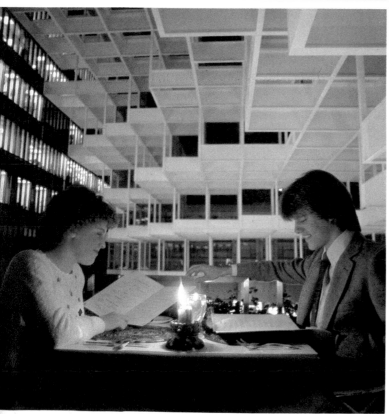

Out on a date, Julie studies a menu, selecting items that fit her meal plan. Like other calorie-conscious diners, she must consider how a food is prepared—whether a fish is broiled, say, or fried in fattening oils—to stay within her daily 1600-calorie limit.

A neat stack of low-sugar cookies rests on the left corner of Julie's music stand during morning band practice. She nibbles on the cookies during breaks in the practice to help maintain stable levels of glucose in her blood between breakfast and lunch.

Overcoming illness to lead a full life

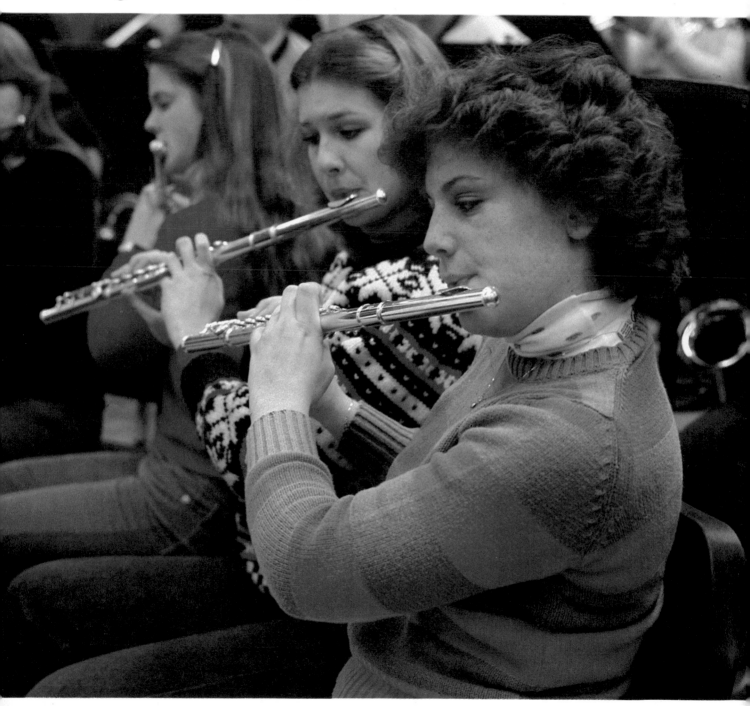

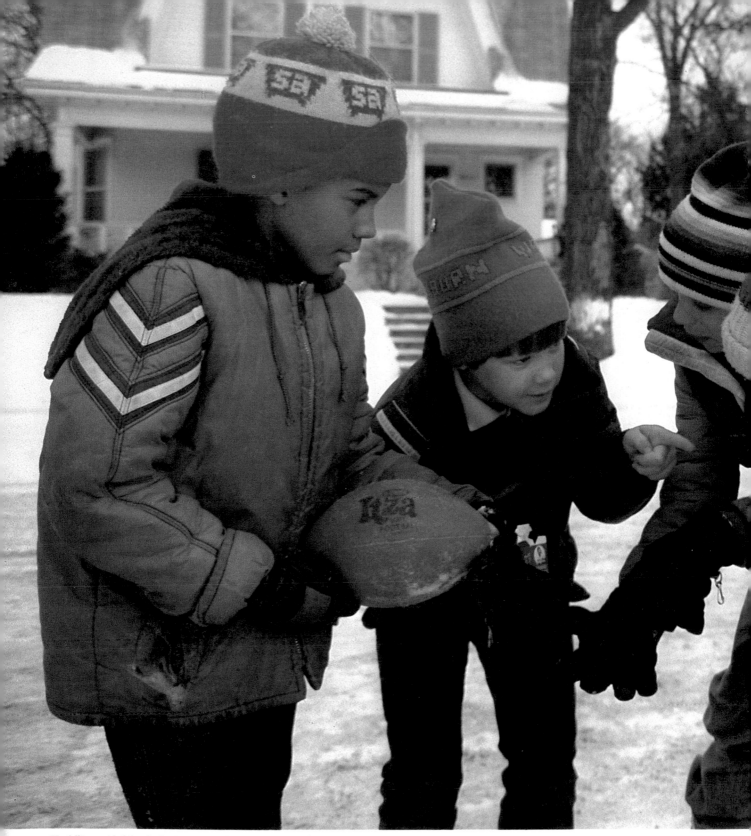

*Huddling with friends during a neighborhood football game,
Michael gives instructions for a play, ready to nibble his required
snack from a box of raisins. Michael carries extra raisins
with him whenever he is out playing to ensure he has a quick
source of carbohydrates close at hand. The snack helps him to
balance his food supply and energy expenditure.*

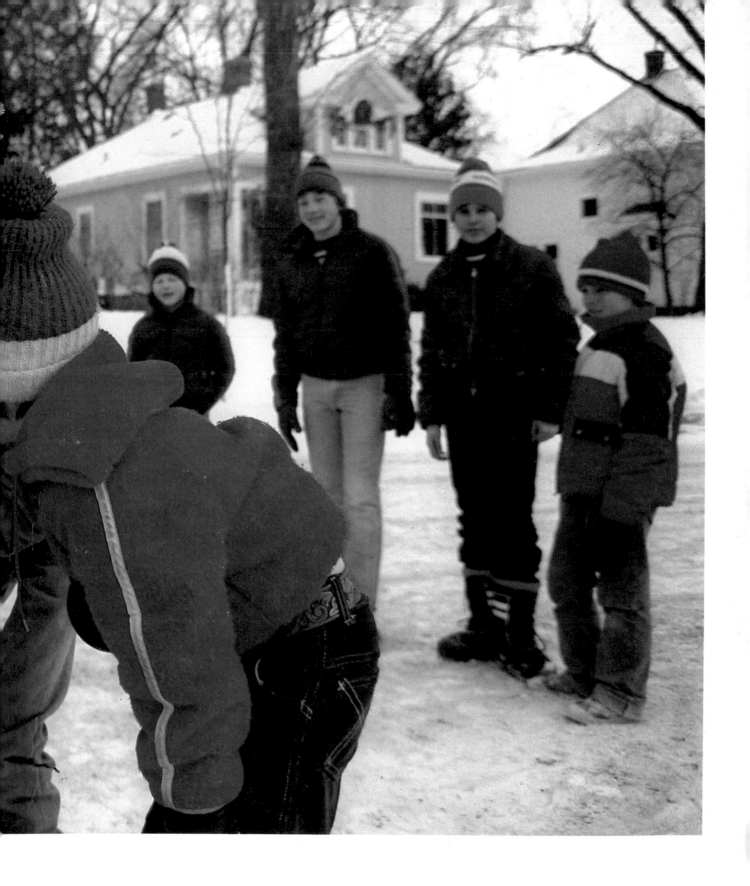

CHAPTER 5

Chemical additives: boon or bane?

Why artificial ingredients are needed
Questions of safety
Breakfast cereals: vitamin-coated candy?
The Chinese-restaurant syndrome
Experts at odds on nitrites, saccharin and dyes
The natural-food alternative

Flour, water and yeast are the basic ingredients in bread; indeed, an excellent loaf can be baked from these ingredients alone. But the recipe for a loaf of supermarket bread is far more complicated. Along with the basic ingredients, there are chemicals—first, calcium propionate; second, a group containing mono- and diglycerides, potassium bromate and ammonium chloride; and another group that includes calcium sulphates, phosphates and carbonates, and niacin, thiamine and riboflavin. This stew of chemicals has aroused a mixture of emotions ranging from bewilderment to mistrust and fear.

The commercial baker would, of course, defend every one of the additional ingredients, or additives (processors learned some time ago that the very word "chemical" tended to dismay their customers, and substituted the more neutral term). The first of the added ingredients keeps the bread fresh for a longer time, the second improves the texture, the third either adds nutrients or restores nutrients that were lost in processing. What is more, the baker would argue that the additives in the bread—or in any other highly processed food, for that matter—are not merely valuable, but necessary. The basis for the larger claim lies in a great revolution in the way life has come to be lived in industrialized countries during the 20th Century.

During the course of the century families have left the farm for the city, and wives have left the kitchen for the office or factory. Kitchen gardens have largely disappeared, and even the minority of the population that grew food for the majority

began to get most of their own foods in shopping expeditions. Giant processing industries in every industrialized nation catered to these new patterns of life with an array of mass-marketed foods, shipped great distances and stored for long periods. More than mere convenience was demanded of these foods: They had to look good and taste good, they had to be safe to eat, however far they had traveled or how long they had been stored, and they had to be uniform in appearance, taste and quality, wherever and whenever they were sold. Enter the additives, which promised—and largely delivered—all these boons.

In themselves, additives were nothing new. Natural additives are almost as old as the history of human food. In ancient times people placed cloves in hams to make the meat keep longer (though they did not know it, the reason cloves worked was that they contain a chemical called eugenol that inhibits the growth of bacteria). Renaissance navigators sailed the world over in search of spices that could be used to mask the taste of tainted food. But more sinister additives appeared then and in later years. The 18th Century novelist Tobias Smollett complained that in the London of his time wine was "balderdashed with cider, corn spirit and the juice of aloes."

These additives were adulterants, designed to stretch the wine without changing its taste; similarly, watered milk, which has a bluish color, was whitened with chalk or plaster of Paris. Far worse were true chemical additives, used in the 19th and into the 20th Century, that endangered the health of

The peaks and valleys at right are the surface irregularities of one white crystal of thiamine, a vitamin used to enrich breads and breakfast cereals. The photographer magnified the crystal 300 times actual size and produced colors with special filters.

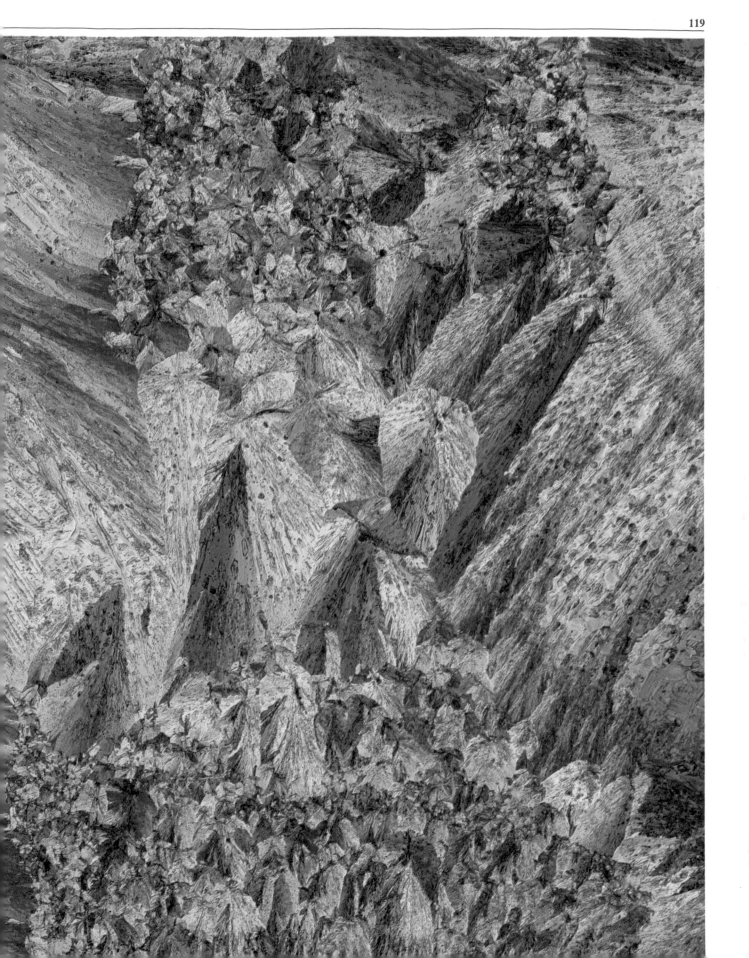

Cream that never saw a cow

Things are seldom what they seem,
Skim milk masquerades as cream.
GILBERT AND SULLIVAN, H.M.S. PINAFORE, 1878

In the good old days England's operetta masters could lament milk substituting for cream. The dry nondairy coffee creamer that is now replacing cream everyplace from airline galleys to home kitchens is a mixture of additives that—except for lactose (a milk sugar), sodium caseinate (a milk protein) and whey—never saw a cow. In most brands, the main ingredients are sweeteners from corn syrup and fats from vegetable oils. Chemical additives supply flavor and color, control acidity, keep the creamer from caking in coffee and make it all mix together. Preservatives prevent the oils from becoming tasteless. Compared with the original, the substitute offers a similar taste, lower price and greater convenience—but may have more undesirable saturated fats than the real butterfat that comes in real cream from real cows.

those who consumed them. Canners, for example, preserved and even heightened the color of green vegetables with copper sulfate—a powerful poison. In the Midlands of England in 1900, brewers sold a beer containing arsenic and sulfuric acid (the acid broke starches down into brewer's sugar; the arsenic came from the ore from which the acid was made). Some 6,000 men and women suffered arsenic poisoning as a result, and 70 died.

What is new about modern additives is their number, their prevalence and a deep concern among the public about their safety. Many of them have been developed recently, so that their long-term impact on health cannot yet be assessed. The number and quantity are astonishing: Well over 2,500 different additives are now used in processed foods; an average diet contains more than 150 pounds of them a year. Over the two decades following 1960, use of additives increased 50 per cent. One result, of course, is the long list of chemicals that now appears on almost every food label or package. After studying one such label on English muffins, the Ameri-

can magazine *The Progressive* commented wryly: "Among the additives in the package is a trace of food." In 1981 *The Times* of London exhibited the label of a "chicken flavoring" for Chinese noodles that contained 10 ingredients—not including chicken, in any form.

Why artificial ingredients are needed

It is easy to understand why such brews arouse bewilderment and alarm. Unfamiliar ingredients in food are a natural cause for suspicion. The purposes of many additives are unclear, so that it is difficult to evaluate the need for them. There are five broad types. In decreasing order of their contribution to health, they are:

● Nutrients. Vitamins and minerals are added to food to make up for possible deficiencies in the ordinary diet, or to replace those nutrients removed in processing. Vitamins are added to milk and margarine to prevent the bone-deforming disease rickets and to prevent blindness, and added to commercially baked breads because some essential vitamins are destroyed in the milling and processing of grain.

● Preservatives. Their role in food is easy to exaggerate—most foods are preserved by canning, freezing and drying. A few preservatives are used in processing, mainly to prevent unappetizing changes in color, flavor and texture when food is exposed to air, or to protect health by blocking poisonous microorganisms. For example, calcium propionate retards the growth of molds on bread, and sodium nitrite in cured meats combats the microorganism that causes the lethal disease botulism.

● Processing aids. They do not make food safer, but they do improve or preserve its taste and texture. Leavening agents help bread and cakes rise; acid-controlling agents regulate tartness. Gelatin thickeners prevent ice crystals from forming in ice cream; glycerin maintains moisture in shredded coconut, marshmallows and candies; lecithin, an emulsifier, keeps the oil and ground peanuts from separating in a jar of peanut butter.

● Flavorings. Sugars and salt make up 93 per cent of the 150 pounds of additives eaten annually by the average individual. Both are natural flavorings; both are unwholesome in the great quantities consumed in the modern diet *(Chapter 4)*. Thousands of other flavorings are eaten in minute quantities, with results that range from innocuous to sinister.

• Colorings. Food dyes are used because food, natural or processed, does not always have the color expected of it. Strawberry jam made from real strawberries is a pale pink; the skin of ripe oranges is often mottled with green; limes are not green, but yellow; butter produced in the months when cows eat hay rather than grass is not yellow, but white. The synthetic colors are potent—in the finished product their presence is generally counted in parts per million—and most are safe. Nevertheless, few additives are more controversial. More than a dozen synthetic food dyes, originally derived from coal tar and long in commercial use, were eventually banned because they may be harmful.

Questions of safety

Though the callous abuses of the 18th and 19th Centuries have all but disappeared, chemical additives are stirring more fear than ever, partly because their failures and hazards are so widely publicized. Hardly a week passes without an announcement that one food additive or another has been accused of causing cancer, birth defects, allergic reactions or disturbing changes in behavior.

Public opinion surveys have shown the effects of such reports: In one poll of more than 1,200 men and women, more than half the group favored the elimination of all artificial colorings from foods, even if that radical move meant that the foods would appear less appetizing. More than 10 per cent of those polled reported that they had recently returned a package to the supermarket shelf when its label showed that it contained additives.

Such alarm is hardly warranted. Of the 2,500 additives used in food, just eight were ordered eliminated in the decade between 1970 and 1980 in the United States. Yet even eight hazardous substances are too many. In 1961 two agencies of the United Nations—the Food and Agriculture Organization and the World Health Organization—began an international effort to set a limit called the Acceptable Daily Intake on each additive in food. By the late 1970s, Acceptable Daily Intakes

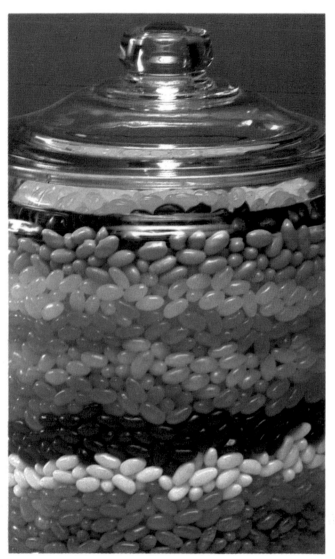

In this rainbow jar of jelly beans, each flavor is identified by a color, a visual cue provided by synthetic food dyes that contribute no taste of their own. Some jelly beans include two colors: The appetizing appearance of watermelon, for example, is suggested by a shell of light pink surrounding a red interior.

were set for more than 400 different additives. These stipulations are recommendations; individual countries, acting on the U.N. studies or on their own research, are left to regulate the use of additives.

Concern is greatest about new additives, and they now are subjected to rigorous tests before their use is permitted. But some additives employed for many years have come under suspicion, and many of them, too, are being tested by methods similar to those applied to new compounds.

Tests on humans are obviously impossible, for ethical and practical reasons. Therefore, the scientists who examine new additives must use laboratory animals. The rigorous United States law requires three animal tests before a new additive can be put on the market.

● The first and most drastic is an acute toxicity test, in which a variety of animals are given massive amounts of the additive to determine the lethal dose—how much is needed to kill them. If the lethal dose is relatively low, the additive will probably never be used in human food.

● A short-term test, performed for 90 days on at least two species of animals, determines the toxic effects of several lower dosage levels.

● A long-term test, also performed on at least two species, lasts two years or more, and shows the effects of lifetime consumption. Over this period some laboratory animals pass through several generations, and the testers can study the effects of the additive on reproduction and on the production of mothers' milk. Lifelong exposure over even a single generation reveals the additive's effects on growth, behavior and death rates.

The validity of animal testing is often challenged. But the obvious and vast differences in the appearances of living things mask fundamental similarities in bodily mechanisms, particularly among mammals. Anything that will make several types of the lower mammals sick will almost certainly make humans sick also; and substances that do not harm the other mammals are unlikely to harm people.

In applying these facts to tests of food additives, scientists deliberately set out to see if a substance can make laboratory animals sick. This essential technique sometimes leads to routines that seem, superficially at least, ridiculous. Some critics, for example, poked fun at tests in which the sweetening additive saccharin was shown to cause cancer in rats, because the animals were fed the saccharin equivalent of 800 artificially sweetened soft drinks a day. No one, of course, could possibly drink that much soda. The huge test dosages make sense, however. If the results overemphasize the dangers of an additive, so much the better—the testing error, if there is any, will be on the side of safety.

The same scientific bias for prudence shows up even more clearly in the human dosage levels that are generally permitted when an additive is eventually approved for commercial use. Typically, the approved level is 1/100 of the highest amount that proved harmless when given to test animals. For example, if test animals show no effects from eating as much as 2,500 parts of an additive per million parts of food, the maximum level allowed by law may be 25 parts per million—the equivalent of .8 ounce per ton of food. Thus, only about .9 ounce of Yellow No. 5, a coloring agent, is added to a ton of pickles.

For additives that may cause cancer, even this wide margin of safety is not enough. No test can ever prove a complete absence of risk, and some cancer-causing substances are potent at concentrations measured in parts per billion. To help prevent the dread disease, many countries place absolute bans on certain additives. Thus, the artificial sweetener called cyclamate has been outlawed in England and Japan. Both cyclamate and saccharin are forbidden additives in France, though their use is permitted in drugs. Red No. 40, a coloring agent and possibly a carcinogen, was never approved for use in England or Canada; Norway and Greece have banned synthetic food dyes altogether.

The most rigorous and sweeping regulations prevail in the United States. In 1958, as part of a law on food additives, the U.S. Congress adopted the so-called Delaney Clause, which prohibits the use of any additive that has been found "to induce cancer in man or animals."

Arguments were brought against the Delaney Clause from the day it was adopted. The legislation singled out additives alone among all the components of human food, although

The crusade for pure food

No matter how tired and hungry and dry,
   The banquet how fine; don't begin it
Till you think of the past and the future and sigh,
   "Oh, I wonder, I wonder, what's in it."

So wrote Harvey W. Wiley, a dabbler in poetry but a chemist of high rank—chief chemist, in fact, of the U.S. Department of Agriculture at the turn of the century. Wiley's doggerel zeroed in on a hot political issue of his day: the purity of food.

For years sporadic press reports had charged that some processors were less than scrupulous in their handling of food; among other things, it was said, they used preservatives that were poisonous. In 1902 Wiley began a series of tests on volunteers *(overleaf)* to see whether the allegations against some of the era's most commonly used preservatives were true. He added minute traces of such substances as borax, benzoic acid and formaldehyde to the otherwise pure food eaten by his subjects. The substances, Wiley

discovered, did indeed produce adverse health effects: Some of the men lost their appetite and became nauseated, and had to be taken off the doctored diets.

Soon Wiley found himself heading a movement to reform the food industry. Muckraking journalists gave the cause momentum. The critical blow was struck by an obscure writer named Upton Sinclair, who in 1906 published a shocking book, *The Jungle,* that told of unsanitary practices in the meat-packing industry. One passage described how packers at a Midwestern plant emptied a vat of meat scraps onto a filthy floor, "then with shovels scraped up the balance" and tossed it in with the good beef.

Although Sinclair had not written the book to aid the pure-food cause—he was a socialist and sought wider political reform—it had that effect: Within three months public pressure forced passage of a tough new law, the first in a series that required proper labeling of food and banned injurious preservatives.

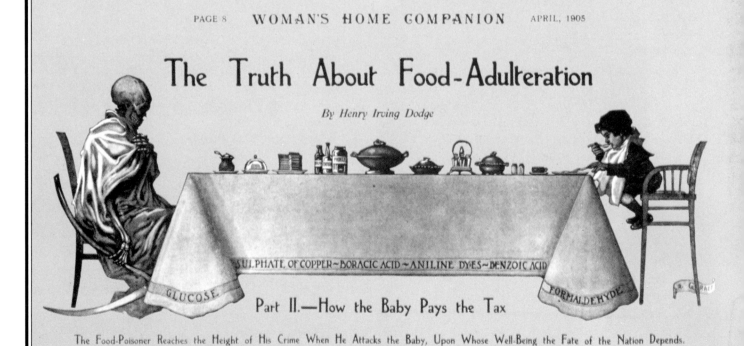

The Grim Reaper sits at one end of a banquet table, an innocent child at the other, in an illustration that accompanied a 1905 Woman's Home Companion article decrying impure food in general and, in particular, the practice of "freshening" milk with such chemicals as boric acid and formaldehyde.

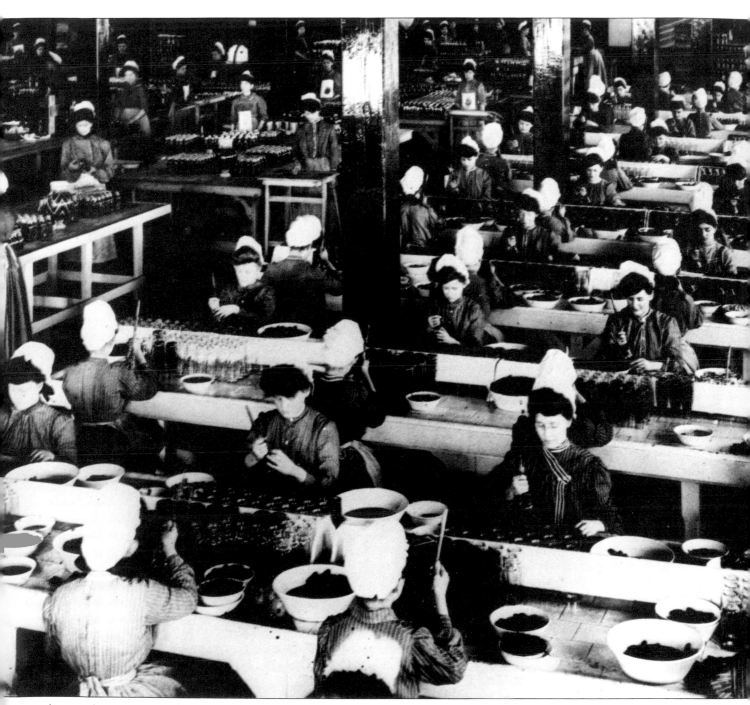

*An exception among turn-of-the-century food processors
in supporting pure-food laws, H. J. Heinz Company practiced
what it preached. Heinz used no artificial ingredients, and
its giant Pittsburgh plant (above) was almost surgically sanitary.
The pickle packers, capped and uniformed, even received
manicures at the company's expense to ensure clean hands.*

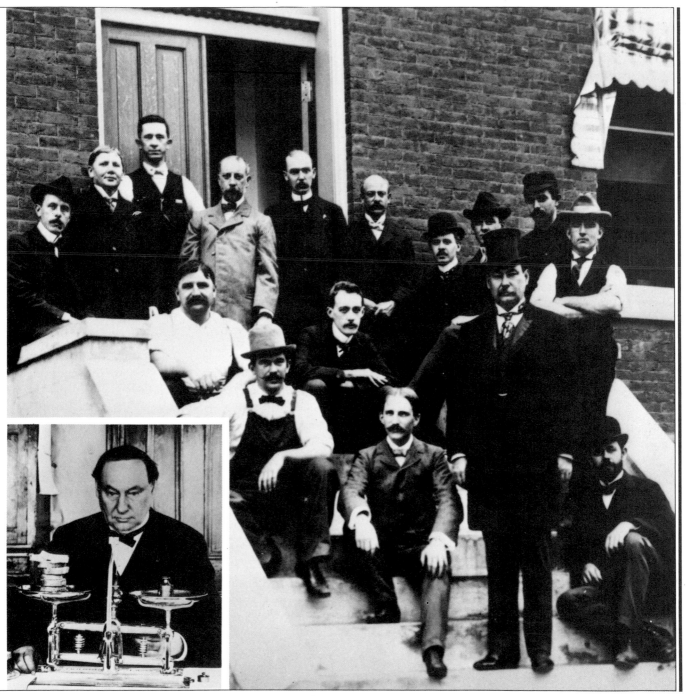

Agriculture Department chemist Harvey Wiley weighs out portions of food for the volunteers testing food additives. Because the first chemical he tested was the preservative borax, members of the press dubbed Wiley "Old Borax."

"Strong, robust fellows with maximum resistance to deleterious effects of adulterated foods" was Wiley's characterization of the food-testing volunteers gathered behind him on the steps of the Agriculture Department's Bureau of Chemistry in the early 1900s. The newspapers, however, called them the "Poison Squad" for eating foods laced with chemicals.

many natural ingredients are known to induce cancer, and others are suspect *(Chapter 4)*. As the science of chemical analysis refined its methods, the detection of infinitesimal and presumably harmless amounts of cancer-causing additives, it was argued, might eliminate a useful and perfectly safe processed food. In addition, the inflexibility of the law prevented regulators from balancing the risks of a substance against its benefits.

The Delaney Clause withstood these assaults. Congress itself addressed the benefit-versus-risk problem by countermanding the Clause when the value of an additive was as evident as its potential danger; thus in 1979 Congress voted to allow temporary continuance of the use of saccharin even though it had clearly caused cancer in experimental animals at high doses—suggesting that its value in helping people control their weight more than compensated for its slight hazards. As for the question of an additive level so low as to be harmless, the National Cancer Institute summed up its answer in a single grim sentence: "We do not know how to establish with any assurance at all a safe dose in man's food for a cancer-producing substance." Under the Clause, action was taken to ban saccharin; 4-4'-methylenebis and flectol-H, two adhesives used in packaging; and diethylstilbestrol and nitrofurazone, two substances used to promote the growth of animals used for meat.

Most American regulations governing additives apply only to new ones, not to those used safely for many years or to "prior-sanctioned" substances, which had been approved for use under earlier laws. The law passed in 1958, for example, exempted 675 additives that had been in regular use before the legislation was adopted. In the language of the law, these substances were a group "generally regarded as safe"—and soon acquired the reassuring nickname of "the GRAS list." To the list, over the years, were added other additives that had been determined by the U.S. Food and Drug Administration (FDA) to be safe.

As it turned out, neither the GRAS-list additives nor the prior-sanctioned group were all that safe. Cyclamate had a secure GRAS status until 1969, when animal tests showed that it caused cancer and it was banned in the United States.

During the 1970s the FDA undertook a full-scale review of all the exempted substances. The review was thorough: It included animal tests, a scrutiny of the medical and scientific literature as far back as 1920 (for one common additive, vitamin A, the reviewers studied 20,000 separate publications) and the verdicts of a panel of experts. Early in 1980 the panel issued its final report to the FDA, covering 415 of the items on the GRAS list. The remaining GRAS substances, spices such as cloves and paprika, used since ancient times, were set aside for separate consideration.

In one respect the report was heartening: All 415 substances were retained on the GRAS list. However, 10 per cent got only qualified approval, and for these, the reviewers said that available information was inadequate for a final evaluation. For a few of these substances—a little over 1 per cent of the reviewed list—GRAS approval was modified: The reviewers recommended that salt and several starches be restricted to levels below their previous use as additives.

Compounds that block metals, molds and malnutrition

Until fears over their safety arose in the 1960s, additives had been considered a miraculous boon of modern chemistry. All are useful in one way or another, and a great many are essential to health. But they can have side effects. The value each confers must be balanced against its potential for harm. Many very useful substances have been avoided simply because they are additives, despite the lack of any evidence that they introduce a health hazard. In some cases—such as those preservatives, nitrites and nitrates—an additive that prevents one disease causes another. In these cases, nice judgment is called for: Is the risk worth the benefit?

Some of the most useful additives are also among the least known. Consider the substance with the mouth-filling name of ethylenediamine tetraacetic acid—mercifully shortened to EDTA. It is not a foodstuff, and neither harms nor helps nutrition. What it does do, and do superlatively well, is form a tight chemical bond with almost any metal. Doctors have long used injections of EDTA to treat cases of acute metal poisoning. The metal and the EDTA, bonded together in the bloodstream, are safely eliminated in urine.

Microscopic particles of metal get into food from processing machinery, and play havoc: They give canned shellfish an unpleasant taste and odor, discolor processed fruits and vegetables, and spoil the oils in margarine, mayonnaise and sandwich spreads. All of these problems are prevented by the addition of EDTA.

Unlike metals, molds occur naturally in food; they are not added by processing or packaging. To retard the growth of molds in bread, processors use a preservative called calcium propionate. It is itself a natural product—about an ounce of Swiss cheese contains enough propionate to protect two loaves of bread—but it is generally produced synthetically. Without propionates, according to one estimate, as much as 10 per cent of the bread in industrialized countries would be needlessly wasted.

Because of the popular wave of protest against all additives, some bakers now omit calcium propionate from their recipes, simply because a loaf without it can be advertised as "free of preservatives." This omission seems counterproductive. As the name implies, calcium propionate adds a supplement of calcium to the diet—minute, but valuable in itself. Far more important is the additive's ability to prevent molds, many of which are dangerous. They can cause infections, skin allergies and a crippling disease called ergotism; mycotoxins, which are by-products of mold growth, are known to cause cancer.

The best known of the mycotoxins is aflatoxin, which develops in nuts, seeds, and grains such as corn and wheat. Heat does not destroy aflatoxin; no known method of processing can effectively remove it from a food. It is carcinogenic in concentrations measured in parts per billion. A jar of preservative-free peanut butter may be safe enough, because U.S. government agencies sample every peanut crop to eliminate contaminated nuts. But grain and flour stored under warm, moist conditions for long periods of time are vulnerable to aflatoxin. Food scientist Thomas H. Jukes of the University of California, Berkeley, has argued that "the use of mold inhibitors as food additives should be expanded for health reasons."

No such fundamental dispute as surrounds preservatives hangs over the additives that supplement food with essential nutrients. Their benefits clearly outweigh their risks. Iodine added to salt has virtually eliminated goiter, vitamin D in milk has made rickets so rare that most medical students never get to study a case, and niacin in breadstuffs has put pellagra under control (Chapter 2).

Breakfast cereals: vitamin-coated candy?
When supplements are used in this way—a single nutrient added to one popular food to solve a single common medical problem—they are almost universally accepted as worthwhile. The additive is one known to be a natural nutrient, and its addition to a single food is unlikely to cause anyone to acquire an excess.

Some such supplements, however, end up in several foods. Iodine is one, found now not only in the salt in the table shaker but also in the plethora of very salty processed foods and in milk from cows given iodized salt. This could lead to an excess. And supplemental vitamins and minerals, each valuable in itself, are added to many processed foods in a variety of combinations, in different amounts and with different objectives. The prime examples of such foods are the modern breakfast cereals, nearly all of which contain a mixture of vitamin and mineral additives. They are also the most controversial. Cereal manufacturers describe their products as the foundation of a balanced diet. Critics call the same cereals little more than vitamin-coated candy.

An ounce of a typical fortified cereal contains about 25 per cent of the recommended daily amount of seven vitamins and one mineral, iron, on the assumption that the breakfast meal should provide about a quarter of a day's nutrients. More recently developed cereals, called supplement cereals, provide much more: up to 100 per cent of the allowances for nine vitamins and iron, with smaller percentages of several other minerals. Such a cereal does indeed amount to something like a crunchy vitamin pill.

Cereals alone, as the manufacturers are careful to point out, cannot supply all of a day's nutrition. Even the most lavishly enriched cereal lacks some of the 40 or more substances needed by humans. In addition, all cereals are low in

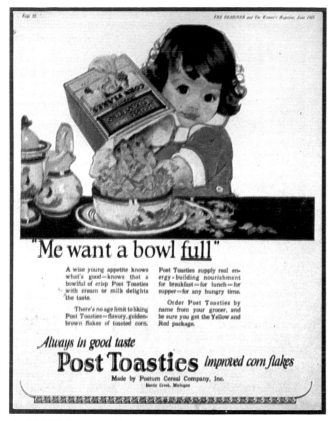

A child fills her cereal bowl to overflowing in a 1923 magazine advertisement for a brand of corn flakes. Little has changed since then in the product or its promotion: Cereals still offer good nourishment and good taste, but their lack of protein and their frequently high sugar content make them less than perfect foods.

fat and contribute little usable protein; the chemical reaction that turns them brown when they are toasted or baked also reduces the amount of an essential protein component, lysine, available to human use. Breakfast cereals also are undesirably rich in salt and sugar—an ordinary cereal consists of about 7 per cent sugar, and presweetened cereals are as much as 54 per cent sugar.

Additional amounts of nutrients are supplied by the milk that is almost always poured into the bowl of cereal—the boxes generally list nutrients in two columns, one for cereal alone, the other for cereal with one-half cup of whole milk. The milk increases the levels of vitamins and minerals, contributes calcium absent from the cereal and supplies additional protein, carbohydrates and fat, making cereal a solid foundation for breakfast. It is only a foundation, however, and most authorities recommend that a cereal-and-milk breakfast also include fruit or juice, along with bread or toast with butter or margarine.

The controversy over the vitamin and mineral supplements in breakfast cereal hinges on their value to nutrition, not their safety. No one seriously believes that they endanger the health of anyone who eats a normal amount of breakfast cereal. But breakfast cereals, along with many other foods, also contain other additives that, like the nutrient supplements, contribute to health but whose potential for harm is still uncertain.

The additives under suspicion include two preservatives, BHA and BHT (acronyms for butylated hydroxyanisole and butylated hydroxytoluene). They are established as positive aids to health. They not only keep fats from turning rancid, but also sustain the strength of the fat-soluble vitamins A and E. They extend the shelf life of a box of breakfast cereal from about four months to a year, and have been used in baked goods, cheeses, meats, vegetables and even chewing gum. What is more, they inhibit the growth of cancer cells in laboratory animals, and some scientists speculate that the fall in the incidence of stomach cancer in the United States may be partly due to the use of BHA and BHT, which were first introduced into food in the 1940s.

But the systematic review of supposedly safe additives

raised questions about these two preservatives. Laboratory rats fed large doses of BHA and BHT developed abnormally large livers. The livers shrank to normal size when the dosages were stopped, and the reason they grew in the first place is still unclear; one theory is that they were not diseased but overactive, because they were producing large amounts of chemical enzymes that help eliminate BHA and BHT from the body. As a result, the safety and continued use of BHA and BHT remain in question. Their benefits as preservatives may not be worth the risk.

The Chinese-restaurant syndrome

Better known than BHA and BHT, but even more mysterious in its action and hazards, is the familiar flavor-enhancer monosodium glutamate, or MSG. It has no flavor of its own, but it somehow intensifies other flavors. Its history is long: Oriental cooks used it for thousands of years in the form of an extract from seaweed, though it was not until 1908 that Kikunae Ikeda, a chemist at the University of Tokyo, identified glutamate as the active ingredient. It later was found to occur naturally in the human body and also in milk, meat and such vegetables as fresh mushrooms and tomatoes. (Some researchers speculated that it was the glutamate in these two vegetables that made them especially valuable as ingredients in otherwise low-flavored stews.)

Inexpensive commercial sources were developed in the 1930s, and processors used MSG not only to make many adult foods taste better but also to give flavor to the bland puréed meats and vegetables of canned or bottled infant foods. Within four decades after introduction of MSG in the United States, some 60 million pounds were consumed by Americans every year.

The safety of MSG was not questioned—it was, after all, a natural substance long used in food in the Orient—until 1968, when a Chinese-American physician, Dr. Robert Ho Man Kwok, called attention to an unusual effect. In a letter to the authoritative *New England Journal of Medicine* he noted, "I have experienced a strange syndrome whenever I have eaten out in a Chinese restaurant." The cause was soon identified as MSG, employed generously in Chinese-American cooking. The symptoms, soon glorified with the title of Chinese-restaurant syndrome, were catalogued: Within 20 minutes after beginning a meal, the victim would experience a burning sensation or numbness in the upper body, sometimes accompanied by chest pain, dizziness, headache, weakness, and nausea and vomiting.

Despite its unpleasant effects the Chinese-restaurant syndrome proved little more than a tempest in a Chinese teapot. For one thing, researchers could not determine its incidence; their estimates ranged from almost 30 per cent in the United States to less than 2 per cent in England. For another, the experience was short-lived—all the symptoms disappeared within four hours. And it turned out that the syndrome attacked only those who ate MSG-laden food on an empty stomach. If the first course of a meal was free of the additive, the syndrome somehow never appeared.

But in 1969, only a year after Dr. Kwok's letter, a far more ominous announcement was made. Dr. John Olney of Washington University in St. Louis reported that, in infant mice, injections of MSG destroyed cells in the hypothalamus, the part of the brain that controls the secretion of hormones. The damage to these young animals occurred even if they were given low doses. "The nerve cells died within hours," Dr. Olney told an interviewer. "We could see this because we dissected the mice. In humans, of course, we can't see if damage has taken place or not."

Dr. Olney's findings did not lead to government action, but they did affect public opinion. Processors no longer add MSG to baby foods. Still, as Dr. Olney himself pointed out in the scientific journal *Neurotoxicology* in 1981, young children continue to be exposed to the additive in such foods as canned soups and vegetables. The future status of MSG remains ambiguous.

Experts at odds on nitrites, saccharin and dyes

The uncertainties that hang over many attempts to link additives with disease may never be fully resolved. Substances such as BHA, BHT and MSG remain suspended in a medical and legal vacuum. On others, the evidence is much less equivocal, and action is taken—yet the problem often is not settled. Additives are banned and then, because of shifts in scientific or public opinion, the bans are rescinded. Many additives are prohibited by law in some countries and permitted in others.

The reasons for this muddle are easy to understand. Every additive serves some purpose that is important to someone, or it would not be used at all. When its benefits, important or trivial, are weighed against its risks, known or suspected, the decision reached depends on who is deciding—and even on when he decides. The difficulty of making a prudent decision in such cases is illustrated by the histories of three different types of additives: the preservatives nitrates and nitrites, the artificial sweeteners cyclamate and saccharin, and the rainbow of dyes that gives processed food its bright colors. All three of these have been linked to the most terrifying of diseases, cancer.

Cured meat gets its pink or reddish color and its distinctive flavor from nitrates or their derivatives, nitrites. Without these preservatives bacon would simply be salt pork, ham would be a heavily salted roast pork, and both would be brown. What is more, the preservatives retard the growth of *Clostridium botulinum* bacteria, which cause a deadly disease, botulism. These bacteria flourish at temperatures between 40° and 140° F. in a damp environment that is free of oxygen. This is a good description of the interior of a cured meat, such as a sausage, at room temperature—and appropriately, the words *"botulinum"* and *"botulism"* come from *"botulus,"* the Latin for "sausage."

In the early 1960s, however, researchers began to discuss a disturbing fact about the nitrites. After food is eaten, the nitrites combine in the body with natural substances called amines, found in saliva and in protein-rich foods, to form chemicals called nitrosamines. Some of the nitrosamines are cancer-causing agents. In 1974 scientists found that one of the most potent of the nitrosamines apparently forms in crisply fried bacon, though not in raw bacon or even in bacon cooked in a microwave oven. Then in 1978, when a study by Paul Newberne of the Massachusetts Institute of Technology indicated that nitrites alone could cause cancer, the United States government made plans to remove them as additives.

Food processors understandably objected to a change that affected the appeal and keeping qualities of their products. But scientists, too, rose to defend nitrates and nitrites. For one thing, they made a strong case against the validity of the Newberne study. In addition, they pointed out that nitrates occur naturally in drinking water and in spinach, beets and a host of other vegetables; at most, only about 20 per cent come from additives. And only a tiny fraction of the nitrosamines in the body are derived directly from food of any kind; the vast majority are formed from the nitrates of saliva. According to Steven Tannenbaum of the Massachusetts Institute of Technology, "About ten times more nitrite enters the stomach daily from nitrate in saliva than from cured meats; probably thousands of times more nitrite is formed in the intestine than is contributed from the diet." More important, eliminating the small risk from nitrate and nitrite additives would greatly increase the risk of botulism.

In 1980 the FDA and the U.S. Department of Agriculture caved in before this storm of protest—but not entirely. These agencies rescinded their plan to eliminate nitrite as a food additive; in effect, as the journal *Science* put it, the government "abruptly told consumers to forget its warning of two years ago that nitrites posed a risk of cancer." But the government also ordered that nitrites be reduced in some products and eliminated from others, and FDA Commissioner Jere Goyan issued a warning: "Nitrites are not home free by any means. There are still questions, and I'm sure they will eventually be phased out of the food supply because of the nitrosamine problem."

While it was scientists and processors who spoke out against a ban on nitrites, it was the general public who objected to attempts to eliminate artificial sweeteners, widely used by people who must avoid eating sugar. The two major varieties, cyclamate and saccharin, have both been implicated as cancer-causing agents, and candidates for their replacement have caused ailments ranging from diarrhea in humans to brain tumors in rats. Yet despite serious doubts about the safety of saccharin and cyclamate, one or both remain in use in countries around the world.

The first sweetener to be attacked was cyclamate, introduced in the 1950s. In 1969 a long-term animal test by a cyclamate manufacturer showed that bladder tumors developed in rats living on feed containing cyclamate. The United States banned cyclamate; soon afterward, Japan and Great Britain followed suit. Yet the picture remained unclear: Ireland, Austria, West Germany and Switzerland never prohibited its use, and later cyclamate tests did not produce tumors in laboratory animals.

With cyclamate banned in some countries and suspect in others, food manufacturers turned increasingly to saccharin. In the United States alone, its use rose to about seven million pounds a year. Two thirds of all additive saccharin wound up in soft drinks—one third of all children under the age of 10-got it from such drinks or from a similar source in processed food—and as many as 70 million Americans used saccharin on a regular basis.

Saccharin had been in use since 1879. Its safety was not challenged until, in one series of experiments, saccharin pellets implanted in the bladders of laboratory animals increased the incidence of tumors. In 1972, American manufacturers were ordered to add a warning to the labels of saccharin containers. Then, in 1977, Canadian researchers at the Health and Welfare Department in Ottawa induced a small number of bladder tumors in the male offspring of pregnant rats by feeding the mothers a diet extremely rich in saccharin. Almost immediately, the Canadian government banned the sweetener, and the United States prepared to do the same.

The outcry that followed in the United States was unprecedented. Dieters, already denied cyclamate and about to lose saccharin, protested that they could not lose weight without the assistance of a nonfattening sweetener; diabetics insisted that for them, saccharin was an absolute necessity, because they could not regulate levels of sugar in their bloodstream. Nutritionists countered that the benefits of the sweetener were primarily psychological and illusory. Since the turn of the century, saccharin had been giving dieters and diabetics the feeling that they were controlling their weight and blood sugar; yet the American population as a whole had become more overweight, and some research suggested that saccharin might actually interfere with blood-sugar regulation.

Adding to the debate, the National Academy of Sciences in the United States issued the results of a review of all the evidence; the Academy concluded that saccharin is a definite, though weak, cancer-causing agent in animals, a probable agent in humans, and a possible cocarcinogen—that is, a substance that stimulates or increases the action of other cancer-causing agents in the body.

During this clamorous, unresolved debate, Congress declared several successive moratoriums on the ban. Canada let its ban stand. Meanwhile, scientists urged the public to reduce its use of saccharin. Dr. Robert Hoover of the National Cancer Institute defined the areas of highest risk. Weighing the evidence of danger against the lack of evidence of benefit, Hoover advised against "any use of saccarin by nondiabetic children or pregnant women, heavy use by young women of childbearing age, and excessive use by anyone."

Even more confusing than the contradictory opinions and regulations about sweeteners is the maze of laws that control the use of synthetic food dyes around the world. Many food dyes are laboratory versions of colorings naturally present in foods; such dyes are not challenged. But others are synthetic in the broad meaning of the term—they are colorings that never exist in nature and can only be created in the test tube. These dyes are carbon compounds made from petroleum by-products. That such carbon compounds can be dangerous has been known since 1775, when Percivall Pott blamed coal soot for the cancer of the scrotum common among London chimney sweeps. Food dyes have long been under suspicion. Yet the laws that affect them vary widely from country to country, and many contradict one another.

Red colorings, the most widely studied food dyes in the world, first aroused concern in the Soviet Union in 1970, when two studies showed that a type called Red No. 2 caused cancer, birth defects and reproductive disorders. However, scientists were not sure that the Red No. 2 employed in the Soviet Union was identical to that used elsewhere, and several experiments were inconclusive. Then a study came up with evidence that the Red No. 2 used in Western Europe and the United States caused cancer in female rats. Male rats seemed unaffected and even the evidence on females was

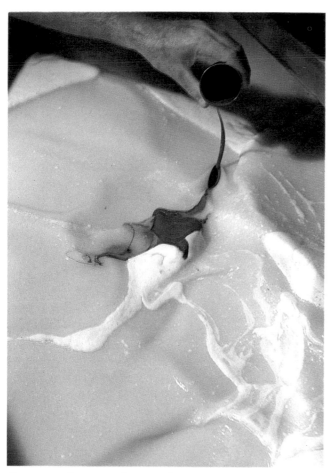

Concentrated carotene dye poured into a vat of oleomargarine gives this white food its familiar yellow color. Produced synthetically or obtained from natural sources—one such source, the carrot, gives it its name—carotene is useful as well as cosmetic: In the body, it is transformed into vitamin A by the liver.

scanty; nevertheless, the United States banned Red No. 2 in 1976, while continuing to permit the use of Red No. 40.

Elsewhere, regulatory agencies took their own courses. France permitted the use of Red No. 2 in caviar, Sweden permitted it in alcoholic beverages; both countries prohibited all other uses. Great Britain and Canada gave full clearances to Red No. 2, but never approved Red No. 40. Subsequent research seemed to confirm their doubts: In one study, mice exposed to Red No. 40 developed cancer at an early age. The only other red dye fully approved as an additive in the United States, Red No. 3, was implicated by studies at the National Institutes of Health in disturbances of the nervous system. And other disorders short of cancer are caused by some of the remaining dyes in the spectrum. Yellow No. 5, for example, causes allergic reactions in 100,000 people in the United States alone, with such symptoms as blurred vision, runny nose, hot flashes and a general feeling of weakness.

Of all the additives, synthetic dyes are the most likely to disappear from processed foods. By 1980, Norway and Greece had banned them altogether, and almost every industrialized country had banned or restricted one or more. These dyes are perhaps the most expendable of additives. Many can be replaced by natural colors or by synthetics that are chemically identical with them; some of these, such as carotene *(left)*, contribute needed vitamins. By contrast, the totally artificial colors, which never existed in nature, offer no nutritional value. Their only virtue is making foods appetizing, although this is a benefit that cannot be overlooked.

When food is the "wrong" color, many people will not buy it. One British grocery chain sold—or tried to sell—raspberry jam and canned green peas prepared without their usual artificial colorings. The sales of these items fell by 50 per cent because the food was so unattractive—the jam was dull brown, the peas gray or yellow.

The natural-food alternative

One result of the hodgepodge of regulation, partial information and misinformation that surrounds processing and additives has been the rejection by some consumers of all processing and all additives. Increasingly people have turned to foods variously termed natural, organic or health foods. In one five-year period during the 1970s the number of American firms specializing in such products quadrupled. Their products, sold in health-food stores or, more often, supermarkets, are expensive, costing 50 to 200 per cent more than their everyday equivalents.

What consumers get for their money is difficult to define. Certainly it is not food completely free of processing. Most health-food users do not drink raw milk, but milk that has been pasteurized to prevent the growth of dangerous bacteria and enriched with vitamin D. In 1980 the U.S. government proposed a definition of natural food as ''minimally processed'' food that contains no synthesized ingredients, such as coloring or flavoring additives or chemical preservatives. This definition does not say anything about how the food was grown—even though natural-food advocates argue that their products are safer and more nutritious not only for their lack of chemical additives but also for being grown without the aid of pesticides or chemical fertilizers.

Most of these claims do not stand up under close inspection. Organic fruits and vegetables, grown with such natural fertilizers as compost and manure, are no more nutritious than produce grown with synthetic fertilizers—and may be less so. Either way, the plants derive their nutrients from the soil. If the soil is deficient in an essential mineral, the compost or manure from animals or plants raised upon it will be deficient too—but a chemical fertilizer can provide the missing nutrient.

Organically grown produce is not sprayed with pesticides, which can indeed leave poisonous residues, but even so this produce is not necessarily pesticide-free. In one test, the New York State Department of Agriculture and Markets found pesticide residues on 30 per cent of a sampling of organic foods bought in health-food stores (only 20 per cent of the ordinary supermarket foods checked bore such residues). The problem is not one of deception or fraud. Because of the way land has been farmed in the industrialized world, it is now almost impossible to grow food free of pesticides. Most land has at some point been treated with chemicals, and the land of an organic farmer contains traces of pesticides that

may take as long as 10 years to disappear completely. And even then, pesticides sprayed by a neighboring farmer or runoff from the rain that falls on his land can taint the organic farmer's land.

There remains the claim that, after its minimal processing, natural food is more nutritious and safer than its everyday supermarket alternative. This claim, too, is shaky at best. Sea salt sold as a health food has no nutritional advantage over regular table salt, and in its natural state lacks the iodine additive that prevents goiter. Honey, brown sugar and refined white sugar are nutritionally more or less identical; all of them provide little of nutritional value other than calories, and all bring the risk of tooth decay. So-called natural potato chips, with the peel left on and without preservatives, are as high in undesirable fat and salt as ordinary chips. Although most health foods are neither better nor worse than their everyday counterparts, some introduce dangers of their own. Herbal teas, for example, contain literally thousands of chemicals that have never been tested for safety, not even by the conventional tests that are mandated by law for additives. When one such tea, made from sassafras, was tested, it turned out to contain a natural flavoring oil called safrole, which causes liver cancer in rats; in the United States, sassafras tea is now banned.

Most natural foods, of course, are neither hazardous nor undesirable. Exactly the same statement can be made of most additives. It is prudent, whenever possible, to eat a variety of fresh or minimally processed foods rather than heavily processed foods with big doses of additives, because the fresh food is generally more nutritious; it is certainly prudent to limit your exposure to artificial flavors and colors, which have no nutritional value at all. Similar rules of prudence apply to natural foods. If you choose to eat preservative-free food, recognize its risks: The molds that form on bread in two or three days can be far more dangerous than the preservative that would have prevented them. You can be sure that fruits and vegetables, however grown, are reasonably free of pesticides only if you wash or peel them yourself. These are common-sense rules, but knowledge and common sense are the keys to a diet that benefits health.

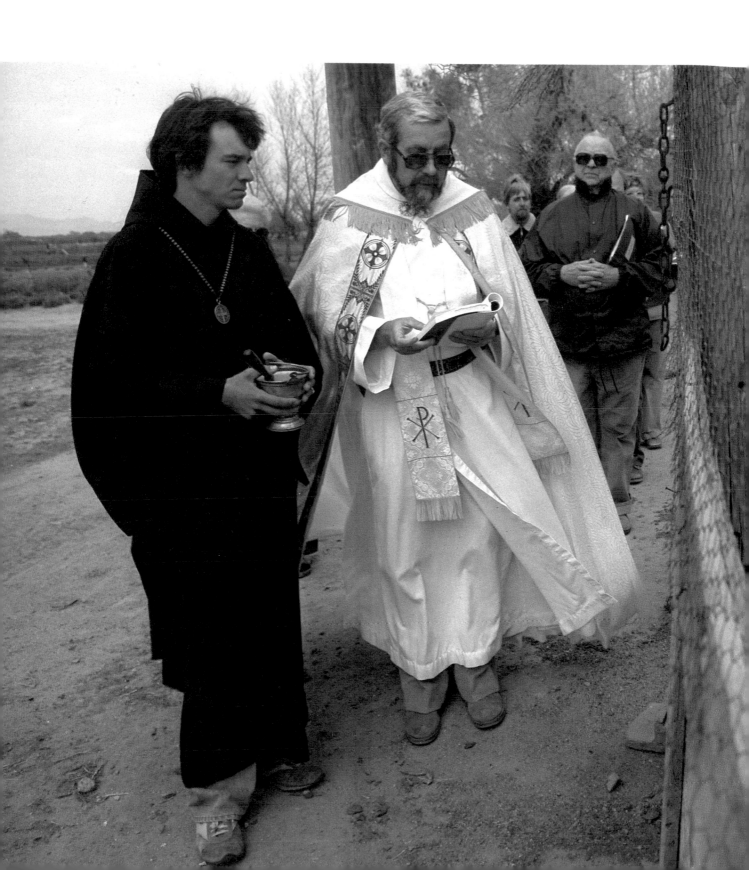

Arizona monks who feast on natural foods

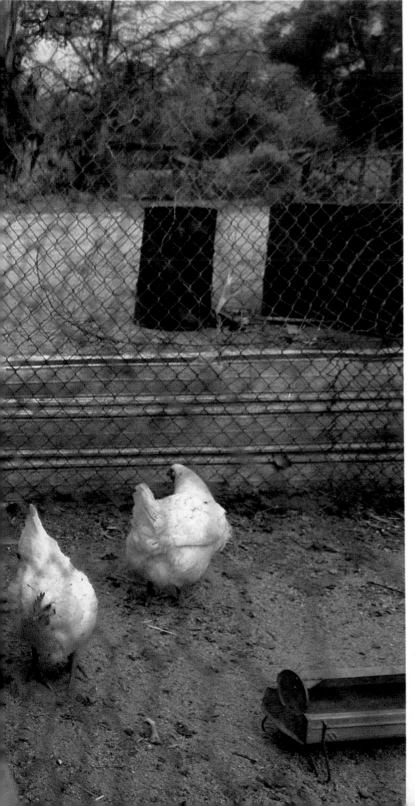

Rare is the family that grows most of the food it eats; rarer still is one that does so largely without resort to pesticides, chemical fertilizers and preservatives, or the other technological aids available to modern farmers and processors. But despite the difficulty of the task, such a family exists: the Benedictine brothers, sisters and lay communicants who live and farm at Holy Trinity Monastery, some 60 miles southeast of Tucson in Arizona's high desert country.

Established in 1974, the monastery puts into practice the teachings of the Sixth Century Roman monk Saint Benedict. He believed that a true Christian community must be totally self-sufficient and that its diet must be wholesome. To the Trinitarians, Saint Benedict's dictum requires that, to the extent possible, foods be grown, preserved and prepared in the traditional ways shown on these and the next 10 pages.

The Trinitarians are guided more by religious belief than by any desire to demonstrate the value to health of organic, or natural, farming and cooking techniques. There is no evidence that their health is better—or worse—than average. The same could be said of their diet. It eliminates certain chemicals—synthetic pesticides, for example—whose safety is challenged; it is generally wholesome, but it must be supplemented by foods bought outside the monastery, including such nutritious staples as milk, whole wheat for bread, and beef. Their acreage could produce more—and slightly more nutritious—food if modern techniques were used: Synthetically fertilized fields are more productive than those enriched naturally, and the foods produced often have a better mix of valuable trace minerals. The Trinitarians' preserving and cooking practices ensure that little is wasted, yet during winter their diet is long on preserved foods and short on the many fresh foods still available in supermarkets—and the supermarket foods are generally superior in nutrients.

Yet the Trinitarians succeed, spiritually and nutritionally. Holy Trinity's 15 or so members grow and prepare about 75 per cent of their own food, and the meals they produce are renowned for wholesome abundance: Midday dinner following Sunday Mass *(pages 144-145)* attracts guests from all over southern Arizona.

Father Louis, Holy Trinity's white-robed prior, leads members in a prayer over two of their 100 chickens—part of the springtime blessing of crops and animals performed on Rogation Days. Fed hormone-free grain, the birds may be less meaty than commercially raised fowl.

Making the most of desert country

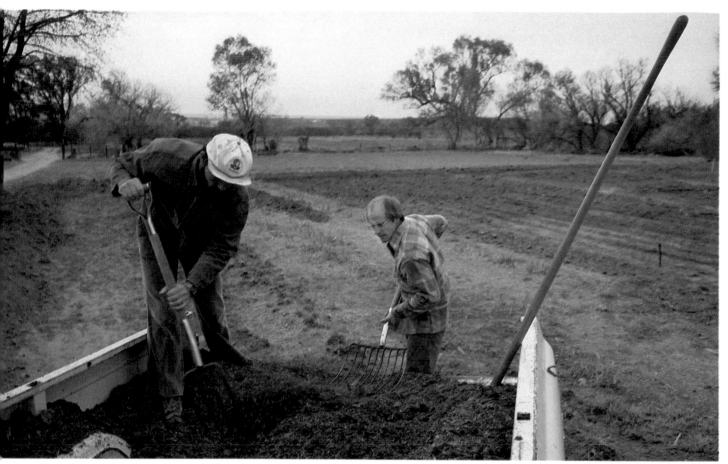

Two of Holy Trinity's lay members dig
into a truckload of silage that they
will spread between rows of vegetables to
stifle weeds and help retain moisture.
The silage will also help to improve the soil
and make the field more productive.

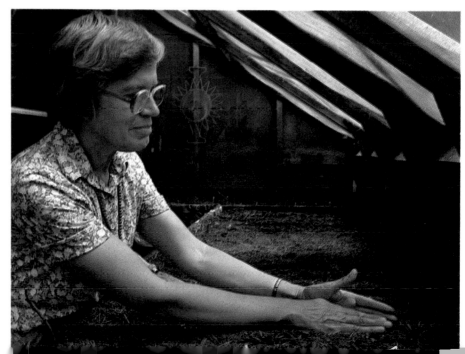

Gently working the soil in a greenhouse
built by the Trinitarians, Sister Ann tends to
a tray full of seedlings. Indoor sprouting
during the off-season is common, ensuring
an earlier supply of nutritious fresh
produce than would otherwise be possible.

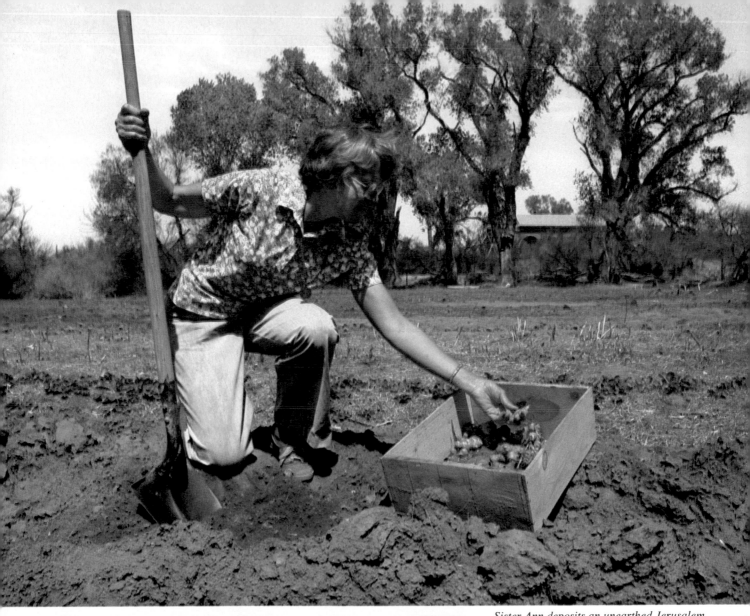

Sister Ann deposits an unearthed Jerusalem artichoke in a wooden box. Organic fertilizer helped produce these healthy tubers, but the plants may contain fewer trace minerals than would a comparable crop grown in chemically fertilized soil.

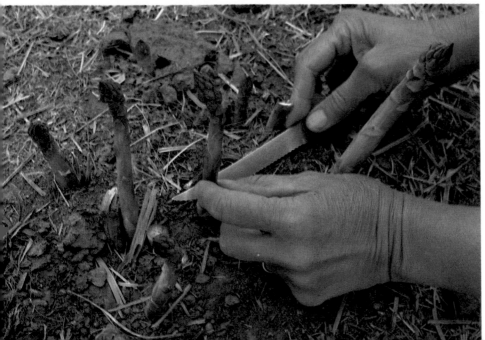

Proceeding stalk by stalk, a communicant goes through the twice-daily ritual of harvesting asparagus, a fast-growing plant. These vegetables were raised free from chemical pesticides, which must be washed off most commercial produce.

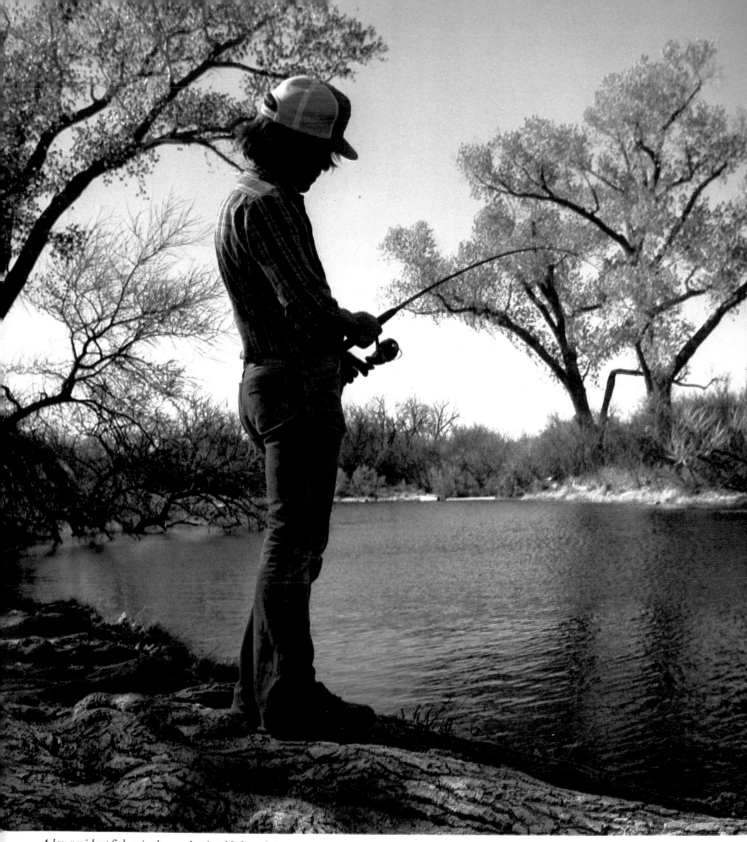

*A lay resident fishes in the productive 10-foot-deep waters
of one of the monastery's two ponds, last stocked with hatchery-
grown bass and sunnies in the late 1930s. The fish provide
the Trinitarians with ample protein, and they do so without the
drawback that accompanies many people's prime source of
the nutrient—the concentrated fat that marbles red meat.*

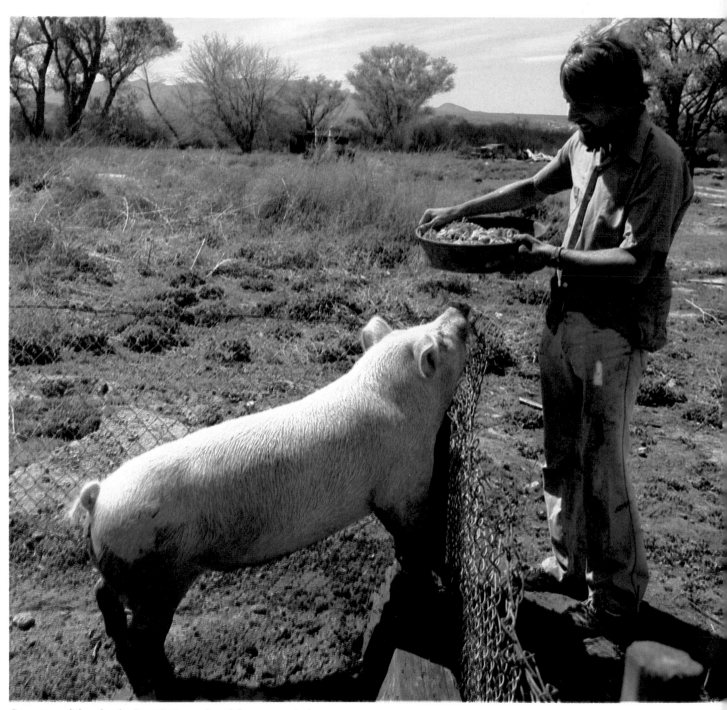

Gary, a candidate for the Benedictine order, delivers a meal of leftovers, kitchen scraps and grain to the farm's lone pig, a four-month-old ''longback'' that will be slaughtered when it reaches 300 pounds. Feeding the pig scraps conserves resources but makes the meat more fatty than it would be if the animal were raised on a regulated diet consisting primarily of grain.

A harvest of wholesome dishes

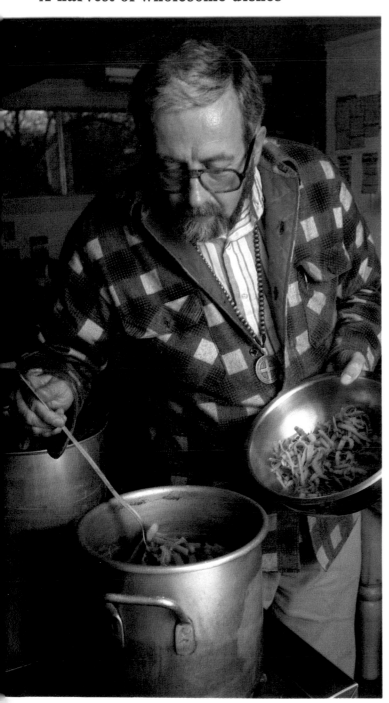

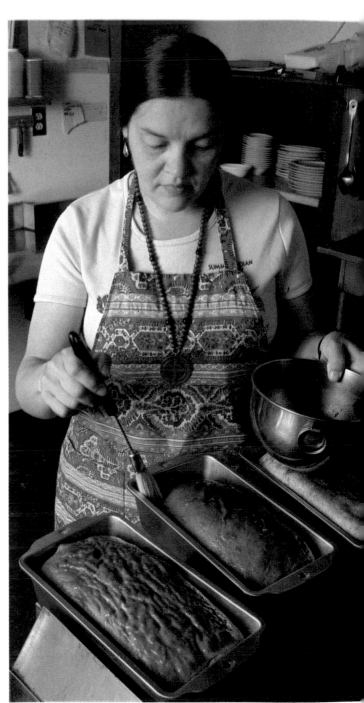

In the monastery kitchen, Father Louis prepares to add carrot skins to a soup that is the repository of the day's vegetable bits and pieces. The next day it will be puréed to create a thick, rich brew, and served as the main course of a meatless meal. This method confers a distinct nutritional advantage—vitamins and minerals in husks and skins are eaten, not thrown away.

Whole-wheat bread, fresh from the oven, is given a final brushing of melted butter by Pat Dawn, a lay member, to soften its crust and improve its taste. But the bread would be better off without it: The butter adds to the loaf's fat content. Although the monastery bakes its own bread, it must buy grain from a nearby market: Wheat is too difficult to grow economically in arid Arizona.

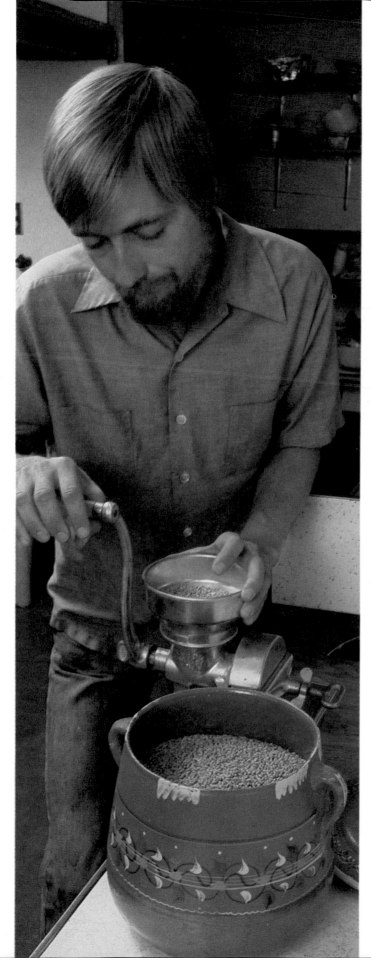

Gary grinds whole buckwheat, bought at the market, for the next day's breakfast porridge. Hand grinding confers no nutritional advantage, but the resultant porridge is certain to be wholesome: Made with unrefined grain, it will include the buckwheat's bran and germ layers, which contain most of the grain's B vitamins: niacin, thiamine and riboflavin.

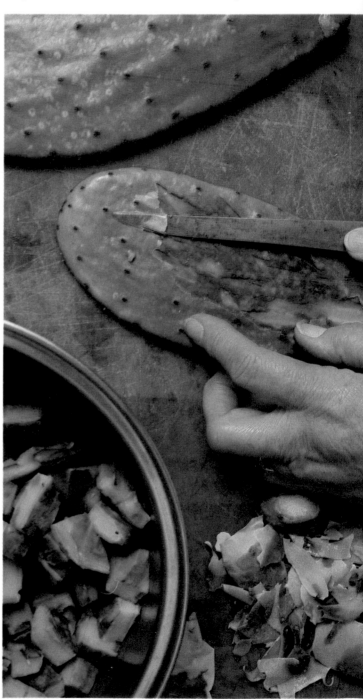

The delicate knife work required to prepare prickly pear, an edible cactus that grows wild in the Southwest, is demonstrated in the close-up above. The plant's spines and outer skin must be pared away so that the desert delicacy can be eaten—an unfortunate sacrifice as the skin contains most of the plant's nutrients. In taste and texture, the peeled plant resembles green pepper.

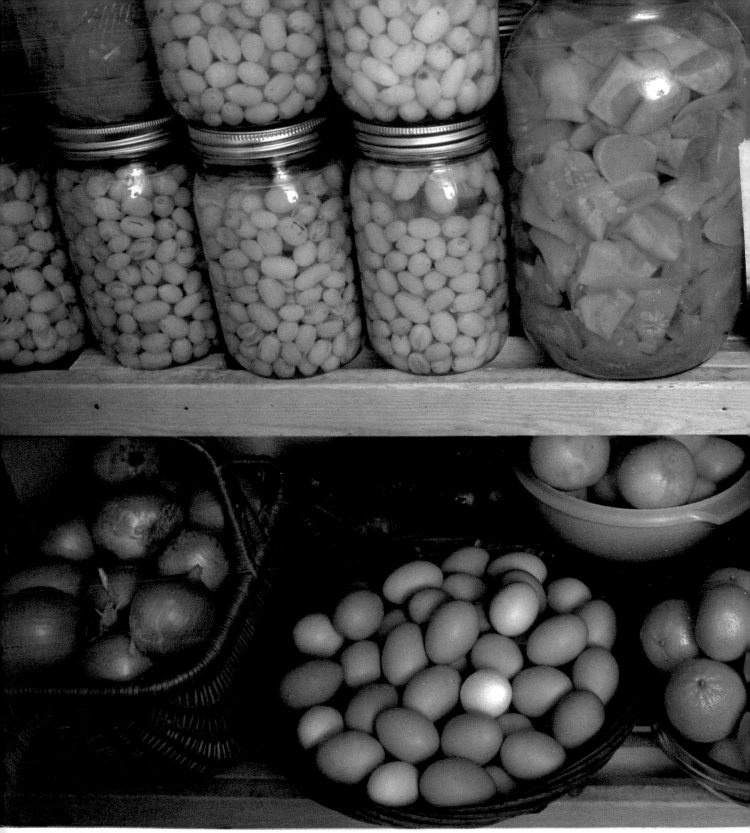

*Jars of pickles, grapes, zucchini and tomato relish—preserves
from last year's harvest—are shelved in a walk-in cooler
above a recent yield of onions, eggs, grapefruit, tangerines and
salad greens. Keeping the jars and fresh foods cool is sound
nutritional practice—temperatures above 80° F. can cause fruits
and vegetables to lose up to 25 per cent of their vitamin C.*

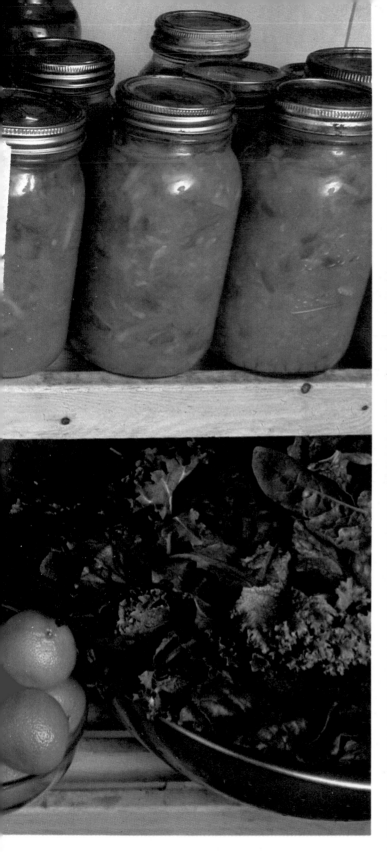

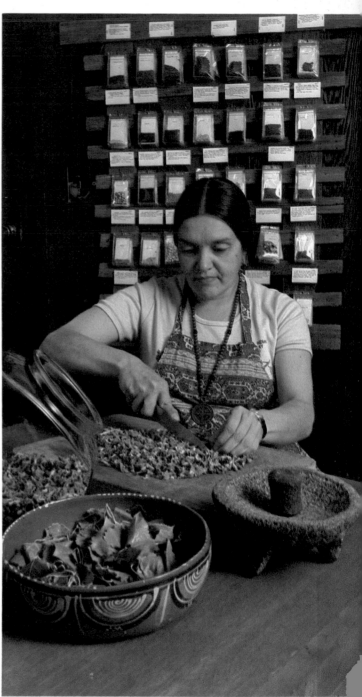

Seated in front of an array of seed packages sold by the monastery, Pat Dawn chops horehound leaves. The bitter mintlike herb is employed to flavor refreshing candies and teas, and often used to soothe sore throats. Unlike horehound, many other herbs are of doubtful benefit: Few have been subjected to laboratory analysis, and some contain chemicals that have been linked to cancer.

A groaning board for Sunday guests

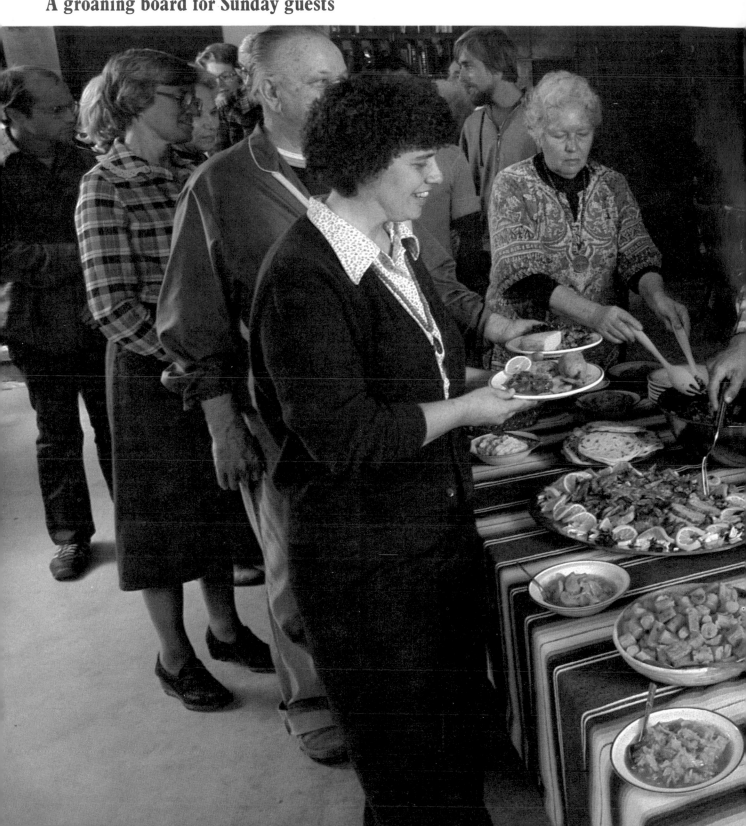

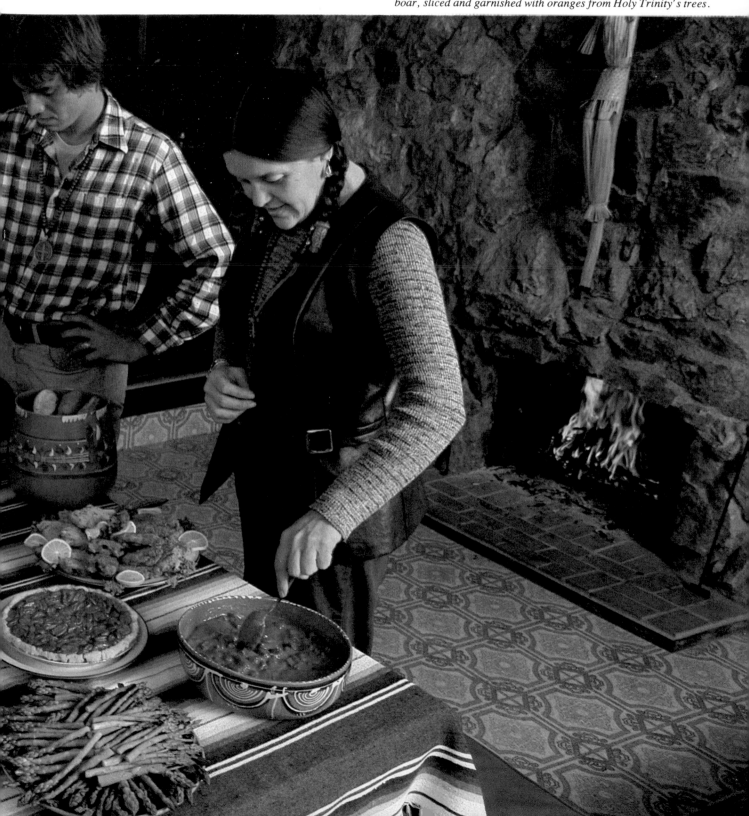

Following Sunday's midday Mass, members of Holy Trinity Monastery and guests gather in the rectory for a well-balanced and largely home-grown feast. Fresh asparagus, carrots and chili made with prickly pear supplement two main courses: fresh bass from the ponds, served with lemon slices, and roast wild boar, sliced and garnished with oranges from Holy Trinity's trees.

CHAPTER 6

Getting full value from the food you buy

Why produce goes bad
Caring for meat, eggs and milk
What you should know about canned and frozen food
How to read a label
Food at home: Handle with care
Cooking for quality

In 17th and 18th Century New England, the last weeks of every winter were a time of privation among the American colonists. A little fresh meat could be obtained from an occasional deer or rabbit skittering across the snowy landscape, but vegetable food was scarce and dismal. Meal after meal consisted of such fare as late-ripening sweet potatoes, dried fruit and the coarsely ground corn called hominy. This lean period, which ended only with the appearance of the first green vegetables of spring, had a grim name of its own: "the six weeks' want."

Today, those New England villages, like towns and cities around the world, enjoy a perpetual harvest. A large supermarket may stock more than 12,000 items. Londoners buy oranges from Mediterranean farms the year round. Lobsters pulled aboard an Atlantic trawler can be bought live at a Chicago fish market 24 hours later. Blueberries, once a short-lived delight of summer, are available anytime in cans. Indeed, some foods, such as lima beans, have become so popular in canned or frozen form that the fresh variety is rarely seen in the bins of a supermarket.

The supermarket is a meeting place of many sciences and technologies. Refrigeration extends the short life span of perishable food. Refrigerated trucks and trains speed chilled food hundreds, even thousands of miles to places where it cannot be grown. Modern techniques of preservation have changed the forms of food, while retaining its flavor and texture to be enjoyed at will, anywhere, anytime.

Maintaining such a safe and steady food supply requires that many foods be canned, dried, frozen, cured or in some way altered from their natural state. Others must withstand the rigors of weeks or months in transit and storage. And changing life styles have dictated that more and more of the food supply be engineered for convenience as well as content. A host of prepared foods—even synthetic substitutes for entire meals—cater to busy people who eat on the run. The price for this variety, safety and convenience: an inevitable loss of nutritional value. The washing, cutting and heating involved in processing, the shipping and storage under widely varying conditions, and even the handling at home— all rob foods of essential nutrients.

The responsibility for assembling a safe, nutritious diet begins in the supermarket. Making informed choices among more than 12,000 foods calls for knowledge of what they are and how they got there.

Fresh foods are best. But in the modern food distribution system, fresh is more likely to mean unprocessed than newly harvested. Fruits and vegetables in the produce section of the average supermarket may not have seen tree or vine for many months. Those glossy red apples, for instance, may have been hibernating in storage for nearly a year.

Usually, however, the time from farm to table is more like a few weeks. This includes a trip of up to a week in a refrigerated truck or railroad car, unloading and reloading at a regional distribution center, a stint in the warehouse if required by the fluctuations of supply and demand, and a final week or so on the supermarket display counter. During this journey,

This robust soup is exceptionally nourishing just because it is soup. Although many foods lose value between farm and kitchen, cooking methods can preserve what is still there —in soup, nutrients dissolved from solid ingredients are eaten in the broth.

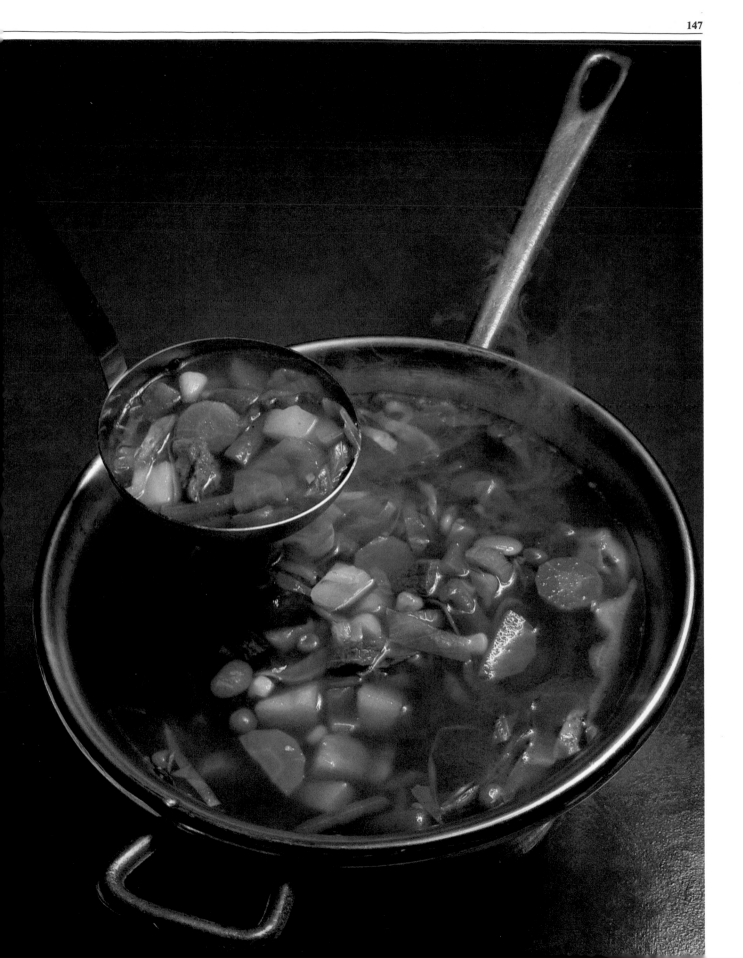

produce is exposed to a variety of conditions that lower nutrient quality. This loss is generally measured in terms of a decrease in the content of vitamin C. Although the other nutrients are important, vitamin C is most widely used as the gauge of nutritional quality in fruits and vegetables for two reasons: It is especially vulnerable to ordinary conditions of shipping and storage, and it is supplied in the diet almost entirely by fruits and vegetables, so that any loss from farm to table is significant.

Why produce goes bad

Even before they are harvested, plants of the same species differ widely in nutritional value. A ripe McIntosh apple has under .0002 ounce of vitamin C. Its lesser-known cousin, the Willowtwig, which is cultivated chiefly in Illinois, contains about .0007 ounce—almost four times as much. Scientists measuring the amount of vitamin A in fresh carrots have found as much as a 21-fold difference between one sample and another. In fact, the nutritional quality of even the freshest produce is affected not only by the breed and maturity of a plant, but also by such factors as the soil and climate that nurtured it.

Harvesting the plant starts processes that lead inexorably to decay and loss of nutrient value. Even after they have been picked, fruits and vegetables remain alive until they are consumed or cooked. They continue to transpire, or evaporate water through their leaves and skins, and to respire, or breathe, by taking in oxygen and giving off carbon dioxide. Once the fruit or vegetable is detached from the parent plant, and thus loses its essential supply of nutrients, both of these normal biochemical processes will result in rapid deterioration if they are not controlled. The leafy green vegetables, because of their large, permeable surfaces, are particularly susceptible to water loss by transpiration after harvesting. With the lost water goes vitamin C.

Refrigeration is the single best method for preventing nutrient loss, because low temperatures retard breathing and evaporation just as they do most chemical reactions. But refrigeration alone is not always sufficient. Some spoilage organisms and enzymes are active at 32° F., the lowest temperature at which fruits and vegetables can be stored without risk of damage from freezing. Some foods, such as tomatoes, bananas and peppers, become susceptible to decay if subjected to temperatures too far above the freezing point. One solution for long-term storage of fruit, especially apples, is hibernation in a controlled atmosphere. The fruit is placed in gastight rooms, and the oxygen is reduced to a level as low as 2 or 3 per cent—those handling the fruit must wear oxygen masks to enter. The low level of oxygen slows respiration and controls the ripening process that causes decay and depletion of nutrients.

Artificially controlled environments are also used to ripen fruit that is most durable when picked green. Bananas, for example, would be destroyed by rot and insects if allowed to ripen on the tree. Instead, they are harvested green and ripened at their destination by exposure to ethylene gas. Tomatoes, which are extremely fragile when ripe, also are picked green and ripened by gassing.

This gassing is not the deception it might seem: Ethylene is a compound used synthetically to make plastics, but it is also a natural ripening agent produced by many fruits and vegetables. But something is lost in picking produce before its time; gassed tomatoes have less flavor than vine-ripened ones, making the latter preferable when available, locally grown, during the summer.

Although any treatment that affects the nutrient quality of fruits and vegetables usually takes place before a customer can see the produce, it may leave visible clues to aid selection. To get the maximum in nutrition, learn a few simple rules for distinguishing truly fresh from slightly spoiled produce. The rules are important for everyone. They are especially important for people who might be harmed if deprived of essential nutrients. The elderly, for example, living on limited incomes, often with missing teeth or ill-fitting dentures that make it difficult to chew high-fiber fruits and vegetables, have a particular need for high concentrations of vitamins and minerals in the produce they eat. Research on the aged has shown that confusion and memory lapses, which are often taken as signs of senility, are sometimes no more than symptoms of malnutrition.

When shopping for fresh produce:
- Avoid produce marked by blemishes, stains or bruises. Such damage hastens decay.
- Choose citrus fruits that are heavy for their size; the juice, in which the nutrients are concentrated, gives the fruit its extra weight.
- Pick fruit for firmness, an indication of maturity that signals maximum development of quality. Ripe apples are taut; pears are best when they have just begun to soften; peaches and apricots should yield slightly to gentle pressure.
- Look for green vegetables that are tender, firm and deep green. If they are wilted, soft or a yellowish color, evaporation has taken away some of their vitamins.
- Select potatoes free of sprouts, which indicate a final stage of maturity leading to decay.

Caring for meat, eggs and milk

Unlike produce, animal products are less likely to lose nutrient value than to decay into inedibility. Until the advent of refrigeration, meat was almost impossible to store during the summer. In *A Year's Residence in the United States,* published in 1818, the English journalist William Cobbett told of an unpleasant encounter with the summer heat of Long Island. Cobbett slaughtered a lamb in August and immediately hung it deep in the shaft of his cool well to keep it fresh. Two days later, he hoisted the lamb to the surface. What he found is reflected in his diary entry for that day: "Resolved to have no more fresh meat till cooler weather comes. Those who have a mind to swallow or be swallowed by flies may eat fresh meat for me."

Laden with moisture and protein, food derived from animals makes an ideal breeding ground for parasites and bacteria that cause spoilage. The only sure way to retard decay and prevent animal fats from turning rancid is to keep all meat, fish and poultry at near-freezing temperatures, which also protect vitamins and minerals.

How well modern refrigeration protects the quality of meat was demonstrated in a 1979 study conducted at Beltsville, Maryland, by the U.S. Department of Agriculture. The USDA scientists selected 18 pork carcasses at a Nebraska meat-packing plant and split them in half. One side of each carcass was shipped directly to Beltsville for analysis. The other halves followed a typical meat-distribution itinerary: They were trucked to California, cut up, and kept for four hours in a supermarket case, closely watched to be sure that shoppers did not walk off with them. Then the supermarket samples, packed in ice, were rushed to Beltsville as luggage on a passenger airliner, and the scientists compared the two shipments for nutritional value. Their decision: The meat shipped to the supermarket had suffered virtually no nutritional loss. "We have to conclude," said Katsuto Ono, a USDA research chemist, "that retailing doesn't affect nutrient composition."

The possibility remains, of course, that meat, poultry or fish may be insufficiently refrigerated anywhere on the long route from slaughterhouse or fishing boat to market. Fish suffers most, because its bacteria, unlike those in meat, flourish even at cool temperatures. To judge freshness and safety, use these guidelines:
- Beef should be cherry-red, firm, and sparsely streaked with cream-colored fat.
- Veal, cut from calves less than three months old, should be a pale or grayish pink.
- The best lamb is light pink in color and plump, with fine, translucent fat.
- Pork should be pale pink, with little fat.
- Poultry meat should be bright and vivid in color; the whiteness or yellowness of its flesh or skin is of no nutritional significance.
- Fish should have bright, transparent eyes, red gills, shiny skin and rich color; when touched lightly, the flesh should spring back. Fresh fish does not have a pungent aroma.

Among the most durable of animal products is the egg. Thanks to human tinkering, eggs are more nutritious than ever before. When a hen is fed a diet rich in vitamins and minerals, it passes the nutrients on in its eggs. Egg farms feed their hens a blend of fresh corn, soybean meal, alfalfa meal, animal fat, calcium-rich limestone, and vitamin and mineral additives, all in pellet or granulated form. The result cannot be matched by a free-ranging hen that chooses its own food.

Catering to the needs of the elderly

At the Pine Street Center in San Francisco's Chinatown, 120 elderly people sit down together every day for wholesome hot dinners of Oriental food—part of a program that, like others around the world, seeks to meet the special nutritional needs of the aged. Because so many old people are relatively poor, live alone and may be unable to cope with shopping and cooking, they constitute a major group of the malnourished in generally well-fed nations. A four-year study in the United States found that more than 80 per cent of those over 65 consumed too few calories, and more than half received too little protein and not enough vitamins.

The San Francisco effort, called Self-Help for the Elderly, is exceptional for its ethnic orientation—large numbers of the city's aged are of Chinese, Filipino or Korean ancestry. Self-Help operates nine centers in different ethnic neighborhoods and supplies traditional dishes to 600 people daily. The Pine Street Center is one of three in Chinatown. The organization also provides home delivery—similar to the "meals on wheels" available in many communities—for the infirm and disabled, but all who can are encouraged to eat at the centers, where they may also receive financial counseling and participate in crafts and games. "One of our aims," said director Vera Haile, "is to get them out of their apartments and together with other people of their age."

The combination of good food and good companionship has proved a smashing success. The Pine Street Center must turn away as many as 30 people a day.

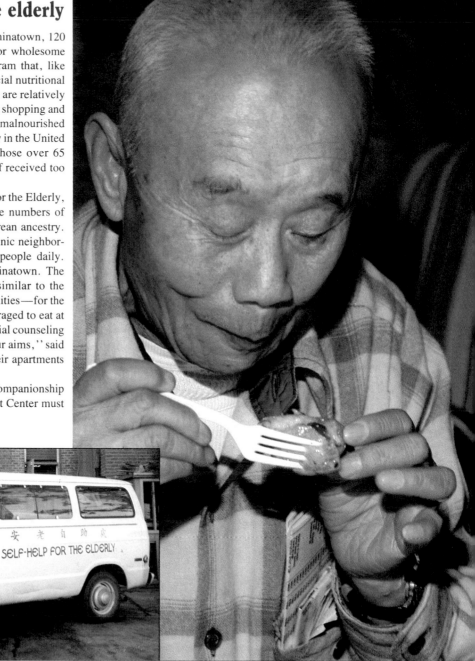

Richard Chung, a 77-year-old member of the board of directors of the Pine Street Center, samples stir-fried chicken— part of the 120 servings of Chinese-style food brought from a caterer to the dining hall by van (left) to provide nutritious, convivial meals for the elderly of San Francisco's Chinatown.

Preparing dishes for the Pine Street Center, cook Shue Kwan Lee transfers freshly made spinach from a large wok to a serving tray. Spinach and mustard greens, also included on Self-Help's menu, are both excellent sources of vitamin A, a nutrient frequently lacking in the diets of the elderly.

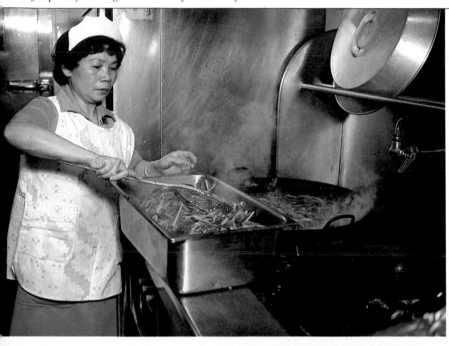

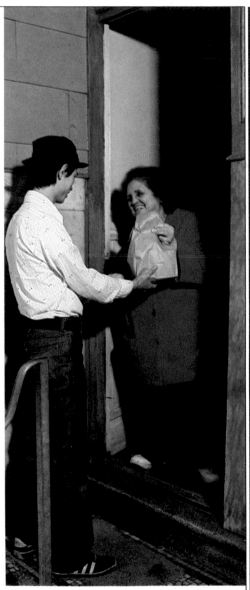

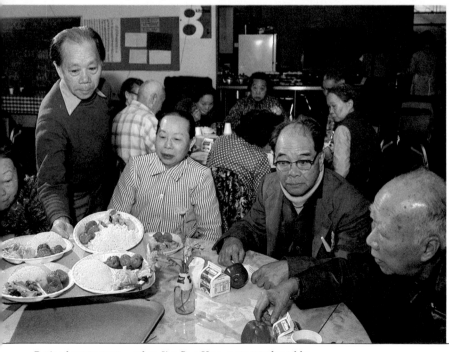

Retired restaurant worker Jim Soo Hoo, now employed by Self-Help, serves up Thursday's meal of braised pork meatballs, cabbage and generous helpings of rice. The Chinese fare that makes up most of the dinner is supplemented by two American-style additions: red apples and low-fat milk.

The Pine Street Center's only non-Chinese member, 72-year-old Sally Weiss, accepts a home-delivered meal from driver Li Wah Kuan. Self-Help provides such service for some 25 participants who are unable to attend the meal centers.

Protected by their shells, eggs do not need the fastidious care that fresh produce does—and it does not matter nutritionally whether the shell is brown or white; the color is determined simply by the breed of the hen. Eggs do require refrigeration because the shells are not completely impervious to bacteria. At 32° F., an egg will retain nearly all its nutrients for about six months; at the higher temperatures of home refrigerators, an egg will keep its fresh flavor and nutritional quality for about five weeks.

By contrast, milk is among the most perishable of animal foods. It is almost always partly processed by pasteurization (heating for 15 seconds at 161° F.), a treatment that kills disease-producing microorganisms but does not destroy the spoilage bacteria. Pasteurization is followed by quick chilling to preserve the milk's flavor.

Pasteurized milk or cream cannot keep in a refrigerator beyond 10 or 12 days. However, much cream and some milk is now being ultrapasteurized—heated for two seconds at 280° F.—so that most spoilage bacteria are eliminated. Treated this way, milk and cream last as long as two months in a refrigerator. Slightly longer heating sterilizes milk so that it keeps at room temperature.

What you should know about canned and frozen food

Like milk, the majority of the foods sold—even those considered fresh—have been processed in some way. Many always have been. The staple of the Western diet, bread, is fresh only by virtue of its brief life. In every other respect it is a processed food, whether baked at home or "made automatically from start to finish," as economist Kermit Bird noted, in "a bakery as large as two football fields. Flour and the other baking ingredients go in one end of a series of integrated machines, disappear from view, and emerge at the other end as fully baked bread ready for cooling, wrapping and delivery." Without counting milk and baked goods, more than half of all American food is processed: canned, frozen or dehydrated. Even in France, where food straight from the farm is considered a birthright, the use of preserved food is increasing.

Processing serves several purposes. It converts foods into usable forms, as by the milling of grain into flour; and it simplifies preparation, as in precooked canned soups or frozen entrées. But its primary function is preventing the microbe growth, enzyme reactions, and chemical changes that cause foods to deteriorate. The goal is to create conditions unfavorable to decay within the food by altering its temperature, moisture content or chemical balance. The most popular processing methods, canning and freezing, involve temperature manipulation. Dehydration—the oldest technique, used to preserve fruits, beans and, in the new form of freeze-drying, instant coffee—simply reduces the moisture content to a level below the minimum at which bacteria breed. Fermentation alters the chemical balance through the action of acid-forming bacteria, yeasts and molds, and in the process turns cucumbers into pickles, cabbage into sauerkraut, and milk into cheese or yogurt. The curing of meat and fish with salt or chemicals such as sodium nitrite also creates a hostile environment for microorganisms and enzymes. It, too, produces foods with a distinctive taste, such as bacon, ham and corned beef.

To varying degrees, all of these methods affect nutrient quality. Chemical additives and fermentation cause relatively little change. In some fermented foods, there actually is an increase in vitamins and protein, which are synthesized by the fermentation organisms. Of all types of processing, heat has the greatest effect on nutrients, but it is also most effective in killing microbes and stopping enzyme reactions. In addition, it destroys antidigestive factors in cereal grains, peas and beans, making it easier for the human body to use the carbohydrates.

The most heat is used in canning, which under some conditions is capable of preventing spoilage for an astonishing time. In 1959, Arnold Bender, professor of nutrition at the University of London, opened a 136-year-old can of veal and a 110-year-old can of mutton retrieved from the Army and Navy Museum. Chemical changes had caused most of the protein in the meat to deteriorate. But Bender reported that "the contents were still sterile," if not very nourishing.

The cans Bender found were exceptional. Most are only "commercially sterile"—they have been heated sufficiently to kill all disease-causing organisms, as well as spoilage bacteria that could grow under normal handling. But if canned goods are kept for a few days at 115° F.—a temperature not uncommon in some storage cabinets—about half will show signs of microbe growth. For safety, all cans more than a year old should be considered suspect.

Unfortunately, the heat that prevents spoilage is also devastating to nutrients, affecting most foods containing little acid, which itself retards the growth of bacteria. Canned tomatoes, which are high in acid, give up only 26 per cent of their vitamin C and none of their vitamin A. Green beans, less acidic, lose 80 per cent of their vitamin C and 22 per cent of their vitamin A in the process. The size of the package also has an influence. Food in a large can is nutritionally inferior to the same food in a smaller can because the big container takes longer to reach the heat of sterilization. A 110-ounce can of peas, supplied to restaurants and institutions and sold in some supermarkets, takes almost twice as long to heat through at the cannery as a 16-ounce can.

Even in frozen foods, heat plays a part. Before vegetables are frozen, they are heated a few minutes, or blanched, to stop chemical activity that freezing does not affect. Unblanched frozen vegetables lose much of their flavor, aroma, color and vitamins within a month.

Despite the brief blanching step, freezing is far easier on nutrients than canning is. In 1963 the U.S. Department of Agriculture compared the vitamins retained by frozen and canned samples of seven vegetables. The frozen samples retained an average of 47 per cent more thiamine, 18 per cent more riboflavin and 25 per cent more niacin and vitamin C.

Freezing, however, does not destroy spoilage bacteria or stop chemical activities to the extent that canning does; it merely holds them in check. If food begins to thaw at any point between the packaging plant and the cooking pot, it loses both nutrients and flavor. Most food thaws at about 25° F., but even lower temperatures can affect the life of frozen foods. A food that will keep perfectly for a year at 0° F., will keep six months at 5°, three months at 10°, and only a day or two at 30°.

Choosing among types of processed foods depends partly on nutrition and partly on expense and taste—frozen peas cost more than canned ones, but are closer to fresh peas in flavor as well as nourishment. Within each type there are huge variations that arise from techniques of the particular processing company and the care—or carelessness—with which its products are handled after they leave the plant. A purchaser cannot, of course, inspect the food itself before buying it. But much can be learned by inspecting the package and its surroundings. They may indicate damage to the contents, reveal the ingredients—including minor ones—and give a date telling when the food has outlived its usefulness.

When checking frozen food at the store, begin with the freezer that contains it. The narrow metal band or tape around the outside of a top-loading freezer case, an inch or two from the top, is the frost line. Below this line, the temperature inside the case is 0° F. or colder, as it must be to keep frozen foods at their best. If packages are piled above the line, avoid them—they may already have begun to thaw. In a front-loading freezer the problem does not normally arise; the outer edges of the shelves on which food is stored lie well within the frost zone. Inside both types of freezers, some stores mount small thermometers; refer to them to be sure that the foods are truly frozen. But the surest clue to quality is the look and feel of the frozen-food package. A limp carton, or one that is wet to the touch, is defrosting. A carton that is stained or caked with frost or ice has definitely thawed and refrozen at some point in its travels. At best, this food will be flawed in taste, texture and nourishment; at worst, it may harbor agents of disease.

Cans, too, can convey signs of mishandling. Look for traces of leakage, a sign of spoilage. Do not buy cans having dents, which may weaken seams and allow bacteria to enter. Bulging is particularly ominous: It is generally caused by microbes that penetrate through a tiny imperfection in the can and stimulate gas-producing reactions.

How to read a label
Processed food seldom disqualifies itself so blatantly. In most cases, the best source of information about canned or frozen food is the label. Embedded in the fine print are useful

data on nutritional quality, age and ingredients—and even what those ingredients add up to, which can sometimes be surprising. A product that calls itself "chicken-flavored noodle soup," for example, probably came from a pot untouched by any chicken. In the United States a can labeled "chicken noodle soup" must contain at least 2 per cent chicken; canned "beef with gravy" must be åt least 50 per cent cooked beef; even "gravy with beef" has a legally prescribed share of meat: 35 per cent.

The word "imitation" generally indicates that a processed food is nutritionally inferior to the natural food it resembles. Imitation strawberry jam, for instance, contains less than 45 per cent strawberries. The choice is not always clear-cut. Imitation mayonnaise may contain less than half the fat and none of the eggs of real mayonnaise—but shoppers who want to reduce fat and cholesterol in their diets may prefer it to the real thing.

Far more important in making dietary choices are the details of a label's list of ingredients. The ingredients are given in the order of their weight, from highest to lowest. Thus, anyone trying to limit his intake of sodium should avoid products that list salt or other sodium compounds among their first few ingredients.

A label may also provide information on nutritional quality, listing the number of calories and the weights of carbohydrates, protein and fat contained in an average serving. Another table may specify, in percentages, how well the helping supplies the recommended allowances of protein, vitamins and minerals.

Finally, a date may be given on a package label or stamped on a can. In many cases the date is embedded in a code meant to be understood only by the manufacturer, but keys to many common codes can often be obtained by writing to government consumer-protection offices. Increasingly, the dates are not coded. This so-called open dating serves two purposes: It tells supermarket staff when to rotate the stock on the shelves and, more important, it gives the shopper an idea of the product's age. Because there is no internationally agreed-upon system of open dating, the procedure varies from place to place.

- A "pack" date indicates when the product was processed. Unless the length of time it can be expected to keep is known, a pack date has little meaning.
- A "pull" date tells the supermarket staff to remove the item from the shelves after a specific point in time, on the assumption that the food will lose much of its nutrient quality or flavor thereafter. The food remains edible for some time after the pull date—but how much time is usually a matter of conjecture for the shopper. Some processors address this problem by printing additional advice on the package, such as "Good for 10 days beyond date stamped."
- A "use-by" date, mandated by law in European Common Market countries since 1981, gives the shopper the clearest possible instructions; it specifies a date beyond which a food should not be eaten. But it also creates the false impression that a food-processing company knows exactly when its product will begin to go bad. In fact no company can ensure that its food will be kept at the correct levels of temperature and humidity as it moves through the stages of shipping, warehousing and retailing. And of course, no open-dating system can take into account the care in storing and handling food receives after it is taken home from the store.

Food at home: Handle with care

After food is purchased, control over its quality passes from the processor and distributor to the consumer, and what happens in a kitchen affects safety and nutrition as much as what occurs in processing and marketing. At home, spoilage is the more important consideration. Nutrient losses will not drastically affect a healthy person; microbes can cause severe illness or even death. Food poisoning is grossly underreported, because its symptoms are often attributed to some unidentified virus. In one recent year, about 11,000 cases of food poisoning were reported in the United States, but public-health officials estimated that the actual total may have been two million.

Food harbors a variety of potentially dangerous organisms. The virus that causes hepatitis can be transmitted by uncooked shellfish taken in polluted waters *(page 155)*. The parasite *Trichinella spiralis,* which commonly infests pork,

The twisted trail of an oyster-borne epidemic

The chart below shows how, in 1960, tainted oysters made their way from the mouth of the Pascagoula River, through the channels of the food industry of southern Mississippi and Alabama, to infect dozens of unlucky shellfish lovers *(black dots)* with hepatitis, a highly infectious liver ailment. The river at the time was carrying untreated sewage that contained hepatitis virus.

The illness hit 17 people who either had tonged the mollusks themselves and eaten their own catch, or had accepted oysters from friends and relatives. Other victims were people who bought oysters in restaurants and markets in Pascagoula, Mississippi, and in Mobile and Troy, Alabama. Those businesses had got oysters

from five different shippers, who in turn had bought from four Pascagoula harvesters—and one in particular. That harvester sold *(bold lines)* to each of the five shippers. One Mobile restaurant was doubly cursed: It purchased oysters directly from the big Pascagoula harvester, then stopped when customers complained of a foul taste, only to buy replacements from an Alabama shipper that had bought some of its oysters from the same source.

All told, 68 people came down with hepatitis. They all recovered, but the incident led health officials to ban oystering temporarily at the mouth of the Pascagoula and then to initiate permanent, year-round inspection of shellfish harvested there.

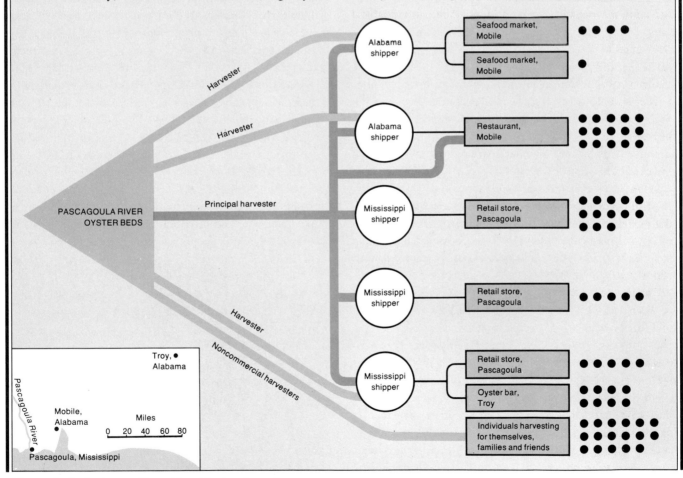

The track of a food-caused hepatitis epidemic—borne by oysters from beds at the mouth of the Pascagoula River, through harvesters and shippers, to consumers in three cities (inset)—is traced above. Each black dot represents one case of hepatitis.

can cause a painful muscle disease, trichinosis. Two poisons produced by molds—aflatoxin, which builds up on such foods as raw peanuts and grains; and patulin, found in apples—are known to cause cancer in animals. But the majority of foodborne illnesses are caused by four classes of bacteria, so common in the environment that government inspections of food-processing plants cannot ensure that food is free of their contamination.

• Salmonella bacteria, found in raw meat, seafood, poultry, milk and eggs, are a leading cause of food poisoning, accounting for some 40 per cent of all cases. Salmonella thrive in foods not cooked thoroughly and in cooked foods kept at room temperatures. They multiply in the intestinal tract and within 48 hours produce diarrhea, abdominal cramps, vomiting and fever. Though seldom fatal, salmonella poisoning can be serious in children under the age of four, the elderly, and the chronically ill.

• *Clostridium perfringens* may survive even in thoroughly cooked meats and gravies in the inactive, harmless form of spores. But if the food is heated and left to stand at room temperature or in a warm oven, the spores rapidly develop into the active form of the bacteria, which multiply in large numbers in the human body and release a toxin that causes gas pains, diarrhea, and occasional nausea.

• *Staphylococcus aureus* produces a toxin in the food itself. A common inhabitant of healthy skin, hair and nasal passages—as well as skin infections—the bacteria multiply in moist meat, poultry, egg dishes, potato salad, cream-filled pastries, custards and gravy kept at room temperature. The toxin released by the staphylococcus withstands later cooking; once swallowed, it causes sudden and violent nausea, vomiting and diarrhea.

• *Clostridium botulinum,* the cause of botulism, releases the most powerful poison known—as little as .0000000035 ounce will kill. Because the toxin is easily destroyed by heat, botulism is a rare disease. Some countries, including England, the Netherlands and Sweden, have gone for years without a single case, Japan averages fewer than five cases a year, and countries such as West Germany and the United States average only 30 to 60 a year. The symptoms of the disease, which appear within 12 to 36 hours, include double vision, impaired speech and difficulty in chewing and swallowing. Anyone who develops this sequence of symptoms should go to a hospital emergency room immediately for treatment with an antitoxin.

The more common forms of bacterial food poisoning call for simpler treatment: Stay in bed and drink plenty of fluids to restore water lost through diarrhea. In most cases, the illness will run its course in a day or two. If symptoms prove severe, though, or persist for more than two or three days, consult a physician.

To avoid food poisoning, protect foods—fresh or processed—against the allies of spoilage: moisture, oxygen and warmth. Even canned goods, the most durable of all, keep better at lower temperatures. Store unopened cans and bottles and packaged dry mixes in a cool, dry place—not in the cabinet above the cooking stove, where warmth hastens deterioration; not in the cabinet beneath the sink, where leaking water can damage dried foods and cause cans to rust. For maximum shelf life, store these foods in a dry place outside the kitchen.

Most fresh foods belong in the refrigerator. The exceptions include potatoes, bananas and hard-rind squash, which keep better in a cool room. Store unripe tomatoes and other fruits at room temperatures until they are ripe, then either eat them immediately or refrigerate them. Because many fruits and vegetables are easily harmed by handling, they retain

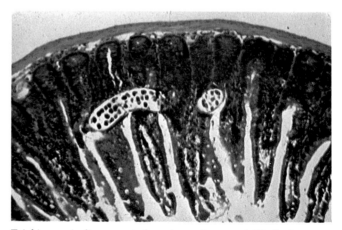

Trichinae spiralis, peanut-shaped roundworms visible in the human intestinal tissue above, cause trichinosis, a dietary disease marked by fever, nausea and muscle pain. Its cause: eating undercooked worm-infested pork. To be safe, pork must be cooked until it is well done—except in Germany, where very strict inspection of pork eliminates infested meat.

nutricnts better if refrigerated unwashed, unstemmed or un-shelled, and loosely packed.

Refrigeration is crucial for animal products. Store meat, eggs and dairy products in the coldest part of the refrigerator. How they should be wrapped is in dispute. Supermarkets employ a plastic film that is semipermeable to oxygen for wrapping their red meat, because freshly cut meat is purplish-red and needs oxygen to turn the bright red that consumers expect. After prolonged exposure to oxygen, however, the meat changes to an unappetizing brownish or grayish red.

This change can be prevented by rewrapping meats with an airtight covering before refrigerating them at home. But tight wraps trap moisture, encouraging a bacterial growth that appears as a slime on the surface of meat. Usually, this growth is not dangerous if the meat is cooked thoroughly, but there is no way of knowing what may be in that mixed population of bacteria. Staphylococcus toxin, for example, would not be destroyed by cooking. In light of this, many experts now advise wrapping meat, poultry and seafood loosely enough to permit some air to circulate inside, keeping the surfaces relatively dry.

The staying power of fresh and frozen foods in the home depends largely on the ability of refrigerators and freezers to maintain suitable temperatures; use thermometers made for the purpose to monitor their operation. Do not keep foods more than a few weeks in the freezing compartment of a one-door refrigerator; temperatures there rarely dip below 10° or 15° F. In a two-door refrigerator-freezer, by contrast, foods will keep in the freezer section for several months. In a separate household freezer, where the ideal temperature of 0° F. can be maintained, foods will keep well for a year. Most refrigerators can maintain the recommended temperature of 40° F., but only frost-free models do so uniformly throughout their interiors. In other types, the temperature is ordinarily lowest just below the freezer unit and highest at the bottom of the storage area.

Even with a refrigerator at a steady 40° F., the rule for maximum quality and safety in fresh foods is to store no more than can be used in three to five days. The most perishable foods are poultry, seafood, ground meat, leftovers, eggs out of the shell and any cooked or uncooked foods containing eggs. Use these perishables within a day or two.

Cooking for quality

Shipping, processing and storage take their toll as food moves from farm to table, but the most destructive stage of the journey is the final one—preparation for eating. Most food poisoning stems from improper handling during cooking and serving. And the steps involved in getting food ready to eat, from trimming and washing to cooking, can be devastating to nutrients.

To overcome the first danger, contamination, follow one ironclad rule anywhere food is served—in the kitchen, at the backyard barbecue, on a picnic, in a boxed or bagged lunch. Keep hot foods hot, cold foods cold, and everything that touches food scrupulously clean.

Between 60° and 125° F., food is in a danger zone, in which bacteria may multiply at a staggering rate, doubling their number as often as every 20 minutes; within seven hours, a single bacterium can produce a colony of more than two million. Foods that spend more than two or three hours within the danger zone may be unsafe to eat. Just above and below the zone some bacterial growth may occur, though at a greatly reduced rate; food is not truly safe, even for short-term storage, unless it is above 140° F. or below 40° F.

Botulism, usually associated with canned foods, struck a 13-year-old California boy who ate a frozen meat pie after it had incubated in an oven for 20 hours. His sister had taken the pie from the freezer and heated it in the oven according to the package directions—20 minutes at 425° F. She then changed her mind about eating the pie, turned the oven off, and left the pie inside. The boy found it the next day, still warm to the touch, and decided to have it for lunch. After a few bites he realized that the pie did not taste right, and he threw it away. But those two or three bites were sufficient to hospitalize him with botulism for eight weeks.

The foods at greatest hazard in the danger zone are essentially the same ones that spoil quickly under refrigeration: meat, poultry, seafood, gravy, stuffing, and mixtures containing eggs or milk. Stuffing is one of the easiest foods to mishandle. Convenience notwithstanding, poultry should never be stuffed until just before roasting; warm stuffing presents a sumptuous feast for bacteria lying in wait within the cavity of an uncooked bird. Pack the stuffing lightly, so that its center will reach a temperature of at least 165° F. during roasting.

Similar hazards exist in many egg dishes. Keep egg salad cold. A cracked egg can be salvaged—but only in dishes that are heated substantially, such as casseroles or baked goods. Do not use cracked eggs to make soft-boiled, poached or scrambled eggs, omelets, meringues, custards or puddings; these dishes are not cooked thoroughly enough to destroy those salmonella bacteria that may have invaded the egg through the crack.

Because of the danger of salmonella contamination, poultry should not be undercooked. To avoid trichinosis, cook pork and pork sausage until they show no sign of pink. Similarly, it is not advisable to sample raw hamburger or cook it exceptionally rare; it can be contaminated by trichinella (if the grinding equipment was used for raw pork), salmonella or parasitic tapeworms.

Reheat leftovers thoroughly—do not merely warm them —because they are frequently mishandled before storage. Cooked foods left sitting on the table after everyone has finished eating, or left to cool slowly on the kitchen counter, may spend several hours in the danger zone. For these foods, correct cooling is as crucial to safety as thorough heating. Refrigerate leftovers promptly and, to be sure they cool as quickly as possible, divide larger quantities into smaller containers, remove stuffing from poultry and carve the meat off large carcasses.

Cleanliness in preparing food may seem simple, but it requires more than ordinary care. A major cause of salmonella poisoning is the inadvertent transfer of bacteria from one food to another. It can occur if a knife or cutting board used for raw meat or poultry is not washed before it comes into contact with other food. Even cooked meat in which salmonella have been destroyed may be recontaminated by an unwashed cutting board.

Fruits and vegetables are the least susceptible to bacterial contamination, but they are the most vulnerable to the loss of nutrients. Ideally most should be consumed unpeeled, uncut and uncooked. For esthetic and culinary reasons, this precept can be applied in only a few cases. But peeling and trimming can be minimized or delayed to salvage the vitamins and minerals concentrated in the outer leaves of vegetables and just under the skins of fruits, roots and seeds. Sliced cucumbers will lose a third of their vitamin C in an hour. Cooked green beans cut into one-inch pieces will retain 52 per cent of their vitamin C; French-style green beans, sliced in lengthwise strips, only 28 per cent. By contrast, potatoes boiled in their skins will retain virtually all their vitamin C, thiamine and other nutrients.

To preserve nutrients, rinse fresh produce no more than is needed to remove dirt, and soak dried peas and beans just enough to soften them slightly. One of the most unnecessary and wasteful practices is washing white rice. The water simply washes away iron and B vitamins added by the processor to replace nutrients lost in milling—a single rinsing removes a quarter of the thiamine in white rice.

As important to nutrition as the preparation of vegetables is the method chosen to cook them. The worst method, unfortunately, is the most common: boiling vegetables for a long time in large amounts of water. That treatment can destroy as much as 80 per cent of the vitamin C and dissolve away other water-soluble vitamins. In one experiment conducted for the United States Army, food chemists compared a batch of cooked cabbage with the water it had been cooked in. Their finding: The water contained more B vitamins than the cabbage. John W. Erdman Jr. of the University of Illinois pointed out that his countrymen "are probably pouring more nutrients down the drain each day than some less fortunate people consume."

Yet nutrient-saving techniques exist in plenty. Despite dire warnings about frying foods, Oriental stir frying is a superior way to prepare vegetables. Frying adds calories to otherwise low-fat foods, but stir frying is so fast it introduces little—and saves nutrients. Even better is the technique of steaming *(page 159),* in which foods do not come into direct contact with water. Whatever method you choose, observe this cardinal rule: Cook vegetables only until they are tender, in just enough fluid to keep them from scorching.

The rules for preparing food seem certain to hold true in the years to come. No one expects food of the future to look or taste markedly different. But it almost certainly will be more packed with nutrients. Scientists are breeding carrots with a higher vitamin A content, corn with less saturated fat and rice with more of the essential amino acid lysine. Already on the market is a super potato with 50 per cent more vitamin C and up to 20 per cent more protein than the other popular varieties.

Future sources of animal protein may include everything from rabbit—an excellent source, still untapped in many countries and low in fat and cholesterol—to a Chilean toad whose meat reportedly tastes like a cross between chicken and lobster. So-called trash fish, until now largely unmarketed because of their gruesome appearances or unappetizing names (the ratfish is just one example) also will become part of the diet, probably under new titles and in minced form. In the Soviet Union and Japan, krill, tiny protein-rich shrimp-like creatures found mostly in the Antarctic, are already being eaten in cheese spreads, meatballs, and stuffings for eggs, fish and dumplings.

As energy costs continue to rise and push up production costs, cans, jars and bottles may become antiques. One possible successor to the can is a retort pouch, made of sealed layers of plastic film and aluminum foil, first used commercially in Japan. Because a typical pouch is only three fourths of an inch thick after filling, pouched food can be sterilized twice as fast as canned food, at a lower cost in energy and with minimal damage to nutrients and taste.

Retort food may be typical of the diet of the future—indistinguishable in content from present-day food but radically different in the way it is processed and packaged. But no radical changes in the food itself seem likely, on the word of Howard Mattson of the Institute of Food Technologists in Chicago. "The basic shape of things we now have on the table," he said, "won't change. We won't be downing little pink pills and calling it supper." ✳

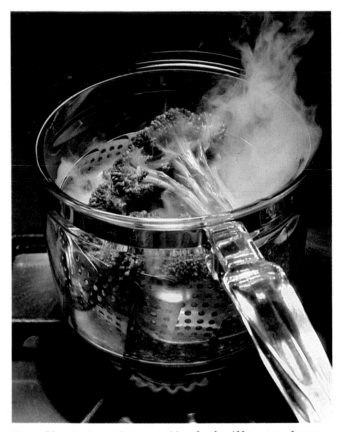

Vegetables retain maximum nutritional value if kept out of water during cooking—when broccoli is steamed, as pictured above (with the lid removed after cooking), it maintains 79 per cent of its content of vitamin C. If the broccoli were immersed in boiling water, it would retain only 33 per cent of its vitamin C.

How to balance a diet

Good food must satisfy a seemingly conflicting set of requirements: taste, economy, calorie content and nutrition. That the requirements are not contradictory is indicated by the tables on the following pages, which characterize 290 common foods and beverages in 10 groups. The listings show that eating right is not merely a matter of counting calories. Nor is it a matter of money—a relatively expensive food such as ham may not deliver as high a nutritional return as the lower-cost sweet potato served with it.

The tables, adapted from *Nutritive Value of Foods,* a 40-page compilation by the U.S. Department of Agriculture, specify the number of calories contributed by each average serving, to aid in the selection of foods that will maintain weight at a desirable level *(Chapter 3)*. For all listings except liquor—which supplies nothing but calories in the form of alcohol—the tables also indicate how big a contribution each serving makes to the daily need for 19 food ingredients. Only the most important ingredients are included: the macronutrients (proteins, fats and carbohydrates), fiber, and 15 key vitamins and minerals. (Details of vitamins and minerals are on pages 43-45.) The amounts of each ingredient are signified by color *(key, lower left, opposite page),* and a star is added to mark those fats that are highly saturated—a chemical type generally considered undesirable—or that contain a large amount of cholesterol.

The tables thus provide an easy way to check whether too little or too much of the important ingredients is provided by the foods ordinarily eaten—and to balance out deficiencies or excesses with other selections.

For all nutrients except fats, sodium and potassium, the higher the intake the better. Most people ingest far too much sodium (in the form of salt); it is believed to play a role in elevating blood pressure. Potassium can build up to toxic levels in those who have heart, kidney or liver problems; however, drugs used to relieve high blood pressure may cause a potassium deficiency and require increased intake of this element. And people who are overweight or suffer from heart or blood-vessel ailments must beware of foods containing large amounts of fats, particularly saturated fats.

Good nutrition can come from a wide variety of foods, detailed in the table that begins at right. It covers 10 categories: beverages, dairy foods, fats and oils, fish and shellfish, fruits and nuts, grain products, meat and poultry, soups, sweets and desserts, and vegetables.

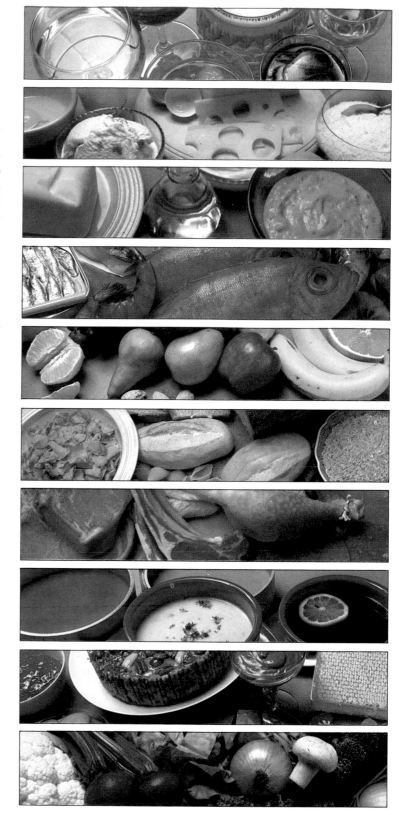

BEVERAGES

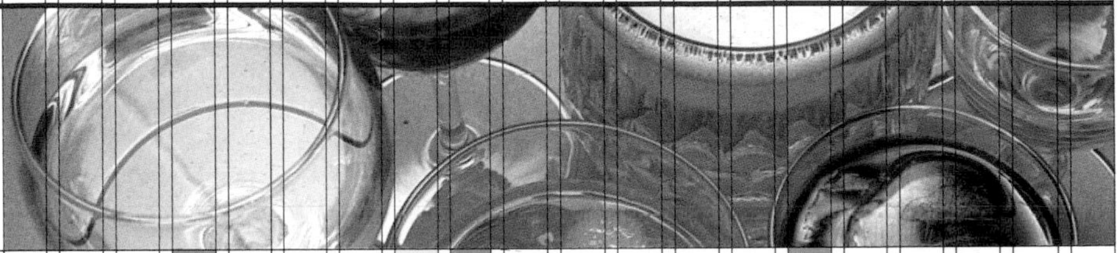

	CALORIES	PROTEINS	FATS	CARBOHYDRATES	FIBER	VITAMIN A	THIAMINE (B_1)	RIBOFLAVIN (B_2)	NIACIN	FOLACIN	VITAMIN B_6	VITAMIN B_{12}	VITAMIN C	CALCIUM	PHOSPHORUS	MAGNESIUM	IRON	ZINC	SODIUM	POTASSIUM
BEER, 12 oz.	150			Average				Small	Average						Average					
COFFEE (with milk and sugar), 1 cup	55			Small																
COLA DRINKS, 12 oz.	145			Large																
FRUIT SODAS, 12 oz.	170			Large																
GINGER ALE, 12 oz.	115			Large																
LIQUOR (86 proof), 1 jigger	105																			
TEA (with sugar), 1 cup	30			Small																
WINES: Dry, 1 glass	85																			Small
Sweet, 1 glass	140			Small																

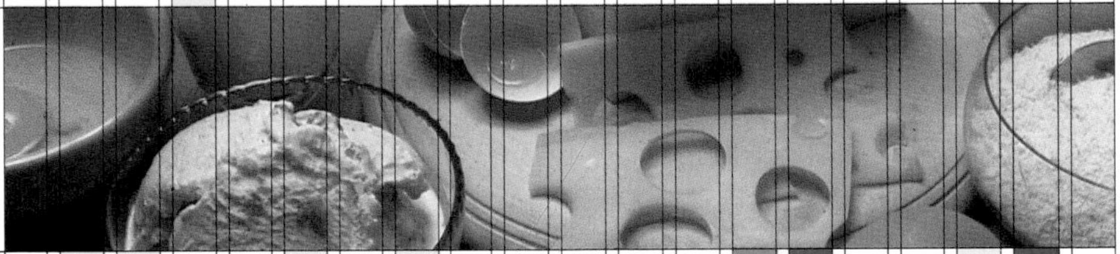

DAIRY PRODUCTS

	CALORIES	PROTEINS	FATS	CARBOHYDRATES	FIBER	VITAMIN A	THIAMINE (B_1)	RIBOFLAVIN (B_2)	NIACIN	FOLACIN	VITAMIN B_6	VITAMIN B_{12}	VITAMIN C	CALCIUM	PHOSPHORUS	MAGNESIUM	IRON	ZINC	SODIUM	POTASSIUM
CHEESE: American, 1 slice	105	Small	★ Small			Small		Small						Average	Large			Small	Large	
American spread, 1 oz.	82		★ Small									Average		Average	Large				Large	
Blue, 1 oz.	100	Small	★ Small					Small				Average		Average	Average				Large	
Cheddar, 1 oz.	115	Small	★ Small			Small		Small				Small		Large	Average				Average	
Cottage (1% fat), ½ cup	82	Average						Average				Average		Small	Average				Large	Small
Cottage (2% fat), ½ cup	102	Average						Average				Large		Small	Average				Large	Small
Cottage (4% fat), ½ cup	117	Average	★ Small												Average				Average	Small
Cream, 1 oz.	100		★ Average			Small													Small	
Mozzarella, 1 oz.	90	Small	★ Small			Small		Small				Small		Average	Average				Small	
Parmesan, grated, 2 tbsp.	130	Average	★ Small					Small						Large	Large				Large	
Ricotta, 1 oz.	71											Small		Small	Small		Average			
Romano, 1 oz.	110	Small	Small					Small						Large	Large				Large	
Swiss, 1 slice	105	Small	★ Small					Small				Average		Large	Average			Small	Small	

Large Amount

Average Amount

Small Amount

Little or None

★ Saturated Fat or Concentrated Cholesterol

	CALORIES	PROTEINS	FATS	CARBOHYDRATES	FIBER	VITAMIN A	THIAMINE (B₁)	RIBOFLAVIN (B₂)	NIACIN	FOLACIN	VITAMIN B₆	VITAMIN B₁₂	VITAMIN C	CALCIUM	PHOSPHORUS	MAGNESIUM	IRON	ZINC	SODIUM	POTASSIUM
CREAM: Half and half, ¼ cup	71		★																	
Heavy whipping, 2 tbsp.	102		★																	
Light, ¼ cup	117		★																	
Sour, 1 tbsp.	25																			
Whipped-cream topping, 2 tbsp.	19																			
EGG: Fried in butter, 1	85		★									Average			Average				Average	
Hard-cooked, 1	80		★									Large			Average		Average			
Large (raw), 1	80		★									Large			Average					
EGGNOG, 1 cup	340	Average	★	Large		Average		Large				Large		Large	Large				Average	Average
ICE CREAM: Regular (11% fat), 1 cup	270		★	Large		Average		Average						Average	Average				Average	
Rich (16% fat), 1 cup	350		★	Large		Average		Average						Average	Average				Average	
Soft, 1 cup	375		★	Large		Average						Large		Average	Average			Average	Average	
ICE MILK, 1 cup	185		★	Average																
MILK: Buttermilk, 1 cup	100			Average				Average				Average		Large	Large				Average	
Chocolate, 1 cup	210		★	Large				Large				Large		Large	Large				Average	
Condensed, 1 oz.	123			Average																
Dried (skim), 1 cup	82											Large		Average			Large			
Evaporated (skim), 1 oz.	11																			
Evaporated (whole), 1 oz.	21																			
Fresh (lowfat, 2%), 1 cup	120		★	Average		Average		Large				Large		Large	Large				Average	
Fresh (skim), 1 cup	85			Average		Average						Large		Large	Large				Average	
Fresh (whole), 1 cup	150		★	Average		Average						Large		Large	Large				Average	
Malted, 1 cup	235		★	Large			Average					Large		Large	Average	Average			Average	Average
Shake (thick chocolate), 1 large glass	355		★	Large	Average	Average		Average				Large		Large	Large				Large	Average
Shake (thick vanilla), 1 large glass	350	Average	★	Large	Average							Large		Large	Large	Average			Large	Large
SHERBET, 1 cup	270			Average										Average						
YOGURT: Low-fat (fruit-flavored), 1 cup	230	Average		Large				Average				Large		Large	Large				Average	Average
Low-fat (plain), 1 cup	145	Average		Average				Large				Large		Large	Large	Average			Average	Large
Nonfat, 1 cup	125			Average				Large				Large		Large	Large					
Whole-milk, 1 cup	140		★	Average				Large				Large		Large	Large				Average	

■ Large Amount

▨ Average Amount

□ Small Amount

□ Little or None

★ Saturated Fat or Concentrated Cholesterol

FATS AND OILS

	CALORIES	PROTEINS	FATS	CARBOHYDRATES	FIBER	VITAMIN A	THIAMINE (B$_1$)	RIBOFLAVIN (B$_2$)	NIACIN	FOLACIN	VITAMIN B$_6$	VITAMIN B$_{12}$	VITAMIN C	CALCIUM	PHOSPHORUS	MAGNESIUM	IRON	ZINC	SODIUM	POTASSIUM
BUTTER (salted), 2 pats	70		★																	
CORN OIL, 1 tbsp.	120		▪																	
LARD, 1 tbsp.	115		★																	
MARGARINE, 2 pats	70		▪			▪													▪	
MAYONNAISE, 1 tbsp.	100		★																	
SALAD DRESSING, 1 tbsp.	65		▪																▪	
VEGETABLE SHORTENING, 1 tbsp.	110		★																	

FISH AND SHELLFISH

	CALORIES	PROTEINS	FATS	CARBOHYDRATES	FIBER	VITAMIN A	THIAMINE (B$_1$)	RIBOFLAVIN (B$_2$)	NIACIN	FOLACIN	VITAMIN B$_6$	VITAMIN B$_{12}$	VITAMIN C	CALCIUM	PHOSPHORUS	MAGNESIUM	IRON	ZINC	SODIUM	POTASSIUM
FISH: Bluefish (baked with butter), 3 oz.	135	▪	★			▪			▪						▪					
Fish sticks (breaded), 3 sticks	150	▪	★									▪			▪				▪	▪
Haddock (breaded, fried), 3 oz.	140	▪	★				▪		▪			▪			▪		▪		▪	▪
Ocean Perch (breaded, fried), 3 oz.	195	▪	★					▪	▪			▪			▪		▪		▪	▪
Salmon (canned), 3 oz.	120	▪						▪	▪			▪		▪	▪				▪	▪
Sardines (canned), 3 oz.	175	▪	★					▪	▪			▪		▪	▪	▪	▪		▪	▪
Tuna (canned in oil), 3 oz.	170	▪	★						▪		▪	▪			▪		▪			▪
Tuna salad, ½ cup	175	▪	★			▪			▪			▪			▪		▪		▪	▪
SHELLFISH: Clams (canned), 3 oz.	45											▪			▪		▪			
Clams (fresh), 3 oz.	65	▪										▪			▪		▪			
Crab meat (canned), 4 oz.	67	▪	★															▪		
Oysters (fresh), 1 doz.	160	▪	★			▪	▪	▪	▪			▪	▪	▪	▪		▪	▪		
Scallops (breaded, fried), 3 oz.	165	▪	▪														▪			
Shrimp (canned), 3 oz.	100	▪	★											▪	▪		▪	▪	▪	
Shrimp (breaded, fried), 3 oz.	190	▪	★						▪					▪	▪		▪		▪	▪

FRUITS AND NUTS

	CALORIES	PROTEINS	FATS	CARBOHYDRATES	FIBER	VITAMIN A	THIAMINE (B$_1$)	RIBOFLAVIN (B$_2$)	NIACIN	FOLACIN	VITAMIN B$_6$	VITAMIN B$_{12}$	VITAMIN C	CALCIUM	PHOSPHORUS	MAGNESIUM	IRON	ZINC	SODIUM	POTASSIUM
APPLE (fresh), 1	80			▧																
APPLE JUICE, 1 cup	120			▧												▧				▧
APPLESAUCE (sweetened), ½ cup	115			▧																
APRICOTS: Dried (uncooked), ½ cup	170			▧	▧	■			▧								▧			▧
Fresh, 3	55			▧	▧	■														
BANANA, 1	100			▧							■									
BLUEBERRIES (fresh), ½ cup	45			▧	■								▧							
CANTALOUPE, ½ melon	80			▧	▧	■							■			▧	▧			▧
CHERRIES: Canned in water (sour), ½ cup	53			▧		▧														
Fresh (sweet), 10	45			▧																
COCONUT (fresh), 1 piece	155		★		■															
CRANBERRY JUICE COCKTAIL, 1 cup	165			▧									■							
CRANBERRY SAUCE, ¼ cup	101			▧																
DATES (fresh), 10	220			▧	■				▧							▧	▧			■
FRUIT COCKTAIL (canned in heavy syrup), ½ cup	98			▧	▧															
GRAPEFRUIT (fresh), ½	50			▧		▧							■							
GRAPEFRUIT JUICE, 1 cup	135			▧									■							
GRAPES (fresh), 10	40			▧																
HONEYDEW MELON, 1/5 melon	100			▧	▧					▧			■							
LEMON, 1	20												■							
LEMON JUICE, 1 cup	55			▧									■							
NUTS: Almonds (shelled), ¼ cup	194	▧	■		■										■	■	▧			
Cashews (roasted in oil), ¼ cup	196		★												▧	■				
Peanut butter, 1 tbsp.	95								▧											
Peanuts (roasted in oil, salted), ¼ cup	210	▧	★		▧				■						■	■			▧	
Pecans (shelled), ¼ cup	203		■		▧		▧			▧						▧	▧			

■ Large Amount

▧ Average Amount

☐ Small Amount

☐ Little or None

★ Saturated Fat or Concentrated Cholesterol

Food	CALORIES	PROTEINS	FATS	CARBOHYDRATES	FIBER	VITAMIN A	THIAMINE (B₁)	RIBOFLAVIN (B₂)	NIACIN	FOLACIN	VITAMIN B₆	VITAMIN B₁₂	VITAMIN C	CALCIUM	PHOSPHORUS	MAGNESIUM	IRON	ZINC	SODIUM	POTASSIUM
Sunflower seeds, 1 oz.	101				●		●	●		●					●		●			●
ORANGE, 1	65			●	●								●							●
ORANGE JUICE (frozen), 1 cup	120			●		●	●						●							●
PAPAYA (fresh), ½ cup	28				●								●							
PEACHES: Canned in heavy syrup, ½ cup	100			●		●														
Fresh, 1	40			●		●							●							●
PEARS: Canned in heavy syrup, ½ cup	98			●	●															
Fresh, 1	100			●	●								●							●
PINEAPPLE: Canned in heavy syrup, ½ cup	95			●									●							
Fresh, ½ cup	40			●									●							
PLUM, 1	30																			
PRUNES (unsweetened, cooked), ½ cup	128			●	●	●											●			●
RAISINS, ½ cup	210			●	●												●			●
RASPBERRIES (fresh), ½ cup	35				●								●							
RHUBARB, ½ cup	190			●	●								●	●						●
STRAWBERRIES: Fresh, ½ cup	28				●								●							
Frozen (sweetened), ½ cup	124			●						●			●							
TANGERINE, 1	40			●									●							
WATERMELON, 1 large slice	110			●	●	●				●						●				●

GRAIN PRODUCTS

Food	CALORIES	PROTEINS	FATS	CARBOHYDRATES	FIBER	VITAMIN A	THIAMINE (B₁)	RIBOFLAVIN (B₂)	NIACIN	FOLACIN	VITAMIN B₆	VITAMIN B₁₂	VITAMIN C	CALCIUM	PHOSPHORUS	MAGNESIUM	IRON	ZINC	SODIUM	POTASSIUM
BAGEL, 1	165			●			●										●			
BARLEY (uncooked), ½ cup	350	●		●												●	●			
BISCUIT, 1	90			●																
BREAD: Pumpernickel, 1 slice	80			●	●														●	
Rye, 1 slice	60			●															●	
White, 1 slice	70			●															●	
Whole-wheat, 1 slice	65			●															●	

Legend: L = Large Amount, A = Average Amount, S = Small Amount, blank = Little or None, ★ = Saturated Fat or Concentrated Cholesterol

Food	Calories	Proteins	Fats	Carbohydrates	Fiber	Vitamin A	Thiamine (B$_1$)	Riboflavin (B$_2$)	Niacin	Folacin	Vitamin B$_6$	Vitamin B$_{12}$	Vitamin C	Calcium	Phosphorus	Magnesium	Iron	Zinc	Sodium	Potassium
BREAD CRUMBS, 1 tbsp.	59			S																
BULGAR (canned), ½ cup	123			L	L										A					
CEREALS: Bran flakes, 1 cup	105			L	A	L	L	L	L		A				A		L	A	A	
Corn flakes, 1 cup	95			L		A	A	A	A				A						A	
Farina, 1 cup	105			L										A	A		A			
Oatmeal, 1 cup	130			L	A			A							A		A		L	
Puffed rice, 1 cup	60			S															A	
Wheat germ, 1 tbsp.	25										A									
CORNMEAL, 1 cup	120			L	L		A										A			
CRACKERS: Graham, 2	55			S																
Saltines, 4	50																		A	
FLOUR: All-purpose, 1 cup	420	A		L			L	L	L						A		L			
Buckwheat (light), 1 cup	340			L											A		A	A		A
Cake flour, 1 cup	350			L			L	A	L								L			
Self-rising, 1 cup	440	A		L	A		L	L	L					L	L		L		L	L
Whole-wheat, 1 cup	400	L		L	L		L		L						L	A	L	A		
MUFFINS: Bran, 1	105			L	A										A		A			
Plain, 1	120			L															A	
PANCAKE, 1	60			L															A	
PASTA: Macaroni (al dente), 1 cup	190			L			A		A						A		A			
Macaroni (soft), 1 cup	155			L			A													
Macaroni and cheese (canned), 1 cup	230		★	L										A	A				L	
Macaroni and cheese (homemade), 1 cup	430	L	★	L		A	A	L	A					L	L		A		L	A
Noodles, 1 cup	200			L			A		A								A			
Spaghetti (al dente), 1 cup	190			L			A		A						A		A			
Spaghetti (soft), 1 cup	155			L			A													
Spaghetti and meatballs (canned), 1 cup	260	A	★	L		A	A		A								L		A	
Spaghetti and meatballs (homemade), 1 cup	330	L	★	L		L	A	A	A						A		L		L	L
PIZZA, 1 slice	145			L										A	A				L	
POPCORN: Plain, 1 cup	25																			

■ Large Amount

▨ Average Amount

□ Small Amount

□ Little or None

★ Saturated Fat or Concentrated Cholesterol

	CALORIES	PROTEINS	FATS	CARBOHYDRATES	FIBER	VITAMIN A	THIAMINE (B_1)	RIBOFLAVIN (B_2)	NIACIN	FOLACIN	VITAMIN B_6	VITAMIN B_{12}	VITAMIN C	CALCIUM	PHOSPHORUS	MAGNESIUM	IRON	ZINC	SODIUM	POTASSIUM
POPCORN: With oil and salt, 1 cup	40																			
PRETZELS (thin), 10	235																			
RICE: Instant, 1 cup	180																			
Long-grain, 1 cup	225																			
ROLL, 1	155																			
WAFFLE, 1	210		★																	

MEAT AND POULTRY

	CALORIES	PROTEINS	FATS	CARBOHYDRATES	FIBER	VITAMIN A	THIAMINE (B_1)	RIBOFLAVIN (B_2)	NIACIN	FOLACIN	VITAMIN B_6	VITAMIN B_{12}	VITAMIN C	CALCIUM	PHOSPHORUS	MAGNESIUM	IRON	ZINC	SODIUM	POTASSIUM
BEEF: Corned beef (canned), 3 oz.	185		★																	
Corned-beef hash (canned), 1 cup	400		★																	
Hamburger (21% fat), 3 oz.	235		★																	
Liver (fried), 3 oz.	195		★																	
Roast (partially trimmed), 3 oz.	165		★																	
Steak (partially trimmed), 3 oz.	330		★																	
Stew with vegetables, 1 cup	220		★																	
CHICKEN: A la king, 1 cup	470		★																	
Broiled, ½ chicken	240		★																	
Fried, ½ breast	160		★																	
Pot pie, 8 oz.	545		★																	
CHILI CON CARNE (with beans, canned), 1 cup	340		★																	
LAMB: Chop (broiled), 2 oz.	120		★																	
Leg (roasted, partially trimmed), 3 oz.	235		★																	
PORK: Bacon, 2 medium slices	85		★																	
Chop (broiled, partially trimmed), 3 oz.	305		★																	
Ham (boiled), 2 slices	130		★																	
Ham (roasted, partially trimmed), 3 oz.	245		★																	
SAUSAGES: Bologna, 2 slices	170		★																	
Frankfurter, 1	170		★																	

	CALORIES	PROTEINS	FATS	CARBOHYDRATES	FIBER	VITAMIN A	THIAMINE (B₁)	RIBOFLAVIN (B₂)	NIACIN	FOLACIN	VITAMIN B₆	VITAMIN B₁₂	VITAMIN C	CALCIUM	PHOSPHORUS	MAGNESIUM	IRON	ZINC	SODIUM	POTASSIUM
Pork link, 2	120		★					■											■	
Salami, 2 slices	180	■	★					■			■						■		■	
TURKEY: Dark meat (roasted), 3 oz.	175	■	★					■	■		■	■			■		■	■	■	■
Light meat (roasted), 3 oz.	150	■	★					■	■		■	■			■		■	■	■	■
VEAL: Cutlet, 3 oz.	185	■	★					■	■		■	■			■		■	■	■	■
Rib, 3 oz.	230	■	★					■	■		■	■			■		■	■	■	■

SOUPS, CANNED

	CALORIES	PROTEINS	FATS	CARBOHYDRATES	FIBER	VITAMIN A	THIAMINE (B₁)	RIBOFLAVIN (B₂)	NIACIN	FOLACIN	VITAMIN B₆	VITAMIN B₁₂	VITAMIN C	CALCIUM	PHOSPHORUS	MAGNESIUM	IRON	ZINC	SODIUM	POTASSIUM
CONSOMMÉ, 1 cup	30																		■	
CREAM OF CHICKEN (diluted with milk), 1 cup	191		★	■		■		■						■	■				■	■
CREAM OF CHICKEN (diluted with water), 1 cup	116					■													■	
CREAM OF MUSHROOM (diluted with water), 1 cup	129		★																■	
SPLIT PEA WITH HAM (diluted with water), 1 cup	189	■		■		■	■		■						■				■	■
TOMATO (diluted with water), 1 cup	86			■		■					■								■	■
VEGETARIAN VEGETABLE, 1 cup	80			■		■													■	■

SWEETS AND DESSERTS

	CALORIES	PROTEINS	FATS	CARBOHYDRATES	FIBER	VITAMIN A	THIAMINE (B₁)	RIBOFLAVIN (B₂)	NIACIN	FOLACIN	VITAMIN B₆	VITAMIN B₁₂	VITAMIN C	CALCIUM	PHOSPHORUS	MAGNESIUM	IRON	ZINC	SODIUM	POTASSIUM
BROWNIE (with nuts), 1	85			■																
CAKES: Angel food, 2 oz.	140			■																
Coffeecake, 2 oz.	175		★	■			■								■		■		■	
Devil's food (chocolate icing), 2 oz.	175		★	■															■	
Gingerbread, 2 oz.	150			■													■			
Poundcake, 1 oz.	165		★	■																
CANDY: Caramels, 1 oz.	115			■																
Chocolate, 1 oz.	145		★	■																
Fudge, 1 oz.	115			■																

■ Large Amount

■ Average Amount

□ Small Amount

□ Little or None

★ Saturated Fat or Concentrated Cholesterol

	CALORIES	PROTEINS	FATS	CARBOHYDRATES	FIBER	VITAMIN A	THIAMINE (B₁)	RIBOFLAVIN (B₂)	NIACIN	FOLACIN	VITAMIN B₆	VITAMIN B₁₂	VITAMIN C	CALCIUM	PHOSPHORUS	MAGNESIUM	IRON	ZINC	SODIUM	POTASSIUM
Gum drops, 1 oz.	100			▪																
Hard, 1 oz.	110			▪													▪			
COOKIES: Chocolate-chip, 4	200		★	▪			▪	▪							▪		▪		▪	
Fig bars, 4	200			▪	▪									▪			▪		▪	
Oatmeal (with raisins), 4	235		★	▪			▪							▪			▪		▪	
Sandwich, 4	200		★	▪													▪			
Vanilla wafers, 10	185		▪	▪				▪									▪			
CUSTARD, 1 cup	305	▪	★	▪		▪	▪	▪						▪	▪				▪	▪
DANISH PASTRY, 1	275		★	▪			▪	▪							▪		▪			
DOUGHNUTS: Glazed (leavened), 1	205		★	▪			▪										▪		▪	
Plain (cake-type), 1	100		▪	▪											▪					
GELATIN, 1 cup	140			▪																
HONEY, 1 tbsp.	65			▪																
JAMS, JELLIES OR PRESERVES, 1 tbsp.	55			▪																
MOLASSES: Blackstrap, 1 tbsp.	45			▪										▪		▪	■			■
Light, 1 tbsp.	50			▪													▪			
PIES: Apple, 5 oz.	345		★	▪		▪	▪										▪		▪	
Blueberry, 5 oz.	325		★	▪		▪											▪		■	
Custard, 5 oz.	285	▪	★	▪		▪	▪	▪						▪	▪		▪		■	
Pecan, 5 oz.	550	▪	★	▪		▪	▪							▪	▪		■		▪	
Pumpkin, 5 oz.	275	▪	★	▪	▪	■	▪	▪						▪	▪		▪		■	▪
PUDDINGS: Chocolate, 1 cup	385	▪	★	▪		■	■		▪			▪								
Tapioca, 1 cup	220		★	▪			▪							▪	▪					▪
Vanilla, 1 cup	285		★	▪		▪		■						■	■					▪
SUGAR: Brown, 1 cup	820			▪										▪	▪		■			■
Powdered, 1 cup	385			▪																
White granulated, 1 tbsp.	45			▪																
SYRUP: Chocolate, 1 tbsp.	125		★	▪											▪		▪			▪
Corn, 1 tbsp.	60			▪																
TOASTER PASTRY, 1	200		■	▪		▪	▪	▪	▪	▪							▪		▪	

VEGETABLES

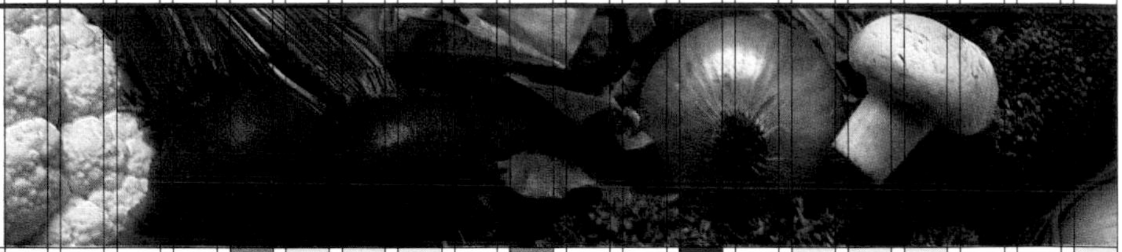

	CALORIES	PROTEINS	FATS	CARBOHYDRATES	FIBER	VITAMIN A	THIAMINE (B_1)	RIBOFLAVIN (B_2)	NIACIN	FOLACIN	VITAMIN B_6	VITAMIN B_{12}	VITAMIN C	CALCIUM	PHOSPHORUS	MAGNESIUM	IRON	ZINC	SODIUM	POTASSIUM
ASPARAGUS: Canned, 4 spears	15				Average	Small	Small	Small		Average			Large		Small	Small	Small			Small
Fresh, 4 spears	10				Average	Average	Small	Small		Average	Small		Large			Small				Small
AVOCADO, ½	195		Large ★	Average	Large	Small	Average	Average	Average		Small		Large		Small	Small	Small			Large
BAKED BEANS (with pork and tomato sauce), ½ cup	155	Small		Large	Large		Average	Small	Average					Small	Average		Large		Average	Average
BEAN SPROUTS, ½ cup	18				Average								Small				Small			Small
BEETS, ½ cup	28			Small	Average					Small			Small			Average				Small
BROCCOLI: Fresh, ½ cup	20				Large	Large	Small	Small		Average	Small		Large	Small	Small	Small	Small	Average		Average
Frozen, ½ cup	25				Large	Large		Small		Average	Small		Large	Small	Small	Small	Small	Average		Average
BRUSSELS SPROUTS: Fresh, ½ cup	28			Small	Large	Small		Small	Small	Average	Average		Large		Small	Small	Small			Average
Frozen, ½ cup	25			Small	Large	Small		Small		Average	Small		Large		Small	Small	Small			Average
CABBAGE: Cooked, ½ cup	15				Average						Small		Large							Average
Raw, 1 cup	15				Average								Large							Small
CARROTS, ½ cup	25			Small	Large	Large					Small		Small			Small				Average
CAULIFLOWER, ½ cup	15				Average						Small		Large							Small
CELERY (diced), ½ cup	10				Average					Small	Small		Small			Small			Small	Small
CORN: Canned creamed, ½ cup	105			Large	Large	Small			Small	Average	Small		Average				Small		Average	
Fresh, 1 small ear	70			Large	Large	Small	Small	Small	Small	Average	Small		Average		Small		Small			Small
CUCUMBER, 6 slices	5												Small							
ENDIVE, ½ cup	5					Average				Large	Small									
GREEN BEANS: Canned, ½ cup	15				Average	Small							Small				Average		Average	
Fresh, ½ cup	15				Average	Small							Average			Small				Average
Frozen, ½ cup	18				Average	Small							Small			Small				Small
KALE, ½ cup	23					Large		Small	Small	Small	Average		Large	Average			Small	Small		Small
LETTUCE: Boston, 2 leaves	3									Small	Small									
Iceberg, 2 leaves	3				Small					Small	Small									
Loose-leafed, 2 leaves	5				Small	Average				Small	Small		Small							

Large Amount

Average Amount

Small Amount

Little or None

★ Saturated Fat or Concentrated Cholesterol

	CALORIES	PROTEINS	FATS	CARBOHYDRATES	FIBER	VITAMIN A	THIAMINE (B₁)	RIBOFLAVIN (B₂)	NIACIN	FOLACIN	VITAMIN B₆	VITAMIN B₁₂	VITAMIN C	CALCIUM	PHOSPHORUS	MAGNESIUM	IRON	ZINC	SODIUM	POTASSIUM
LIMA BEANS, ½ cup	130	░		■	■					░					▒	▒	■		░	■
MUSHROOMS, ½ cup	10				░			▒	░	░										
MUSTARD GREENS (cooked), ½ cup	15				■	■							■	▒			░			
ONIONS (sliced), ½ cup	23																			
PARSLEY (chopped), 1 tbsp.	6												░							
PEAS: Canned, ½ cup	75				▒	■	░										▒		▒	
Frozen, ½ cup	55					■		▒			▒							▒			
PEPPER (sweet), 1	15					■								■						
PICKLE (dill), 1 medium	5																		■	▒
POTATOES: Baked, 1	145				■			▒		▒		░		■		▒	▒				■
Boiled (cooked after peeling), 1	105				■	░				▒				■							■
Boiled (cooked before peeling), 1	90				■	░								■							
French fried, 10 strips	110				■																
Hash-brown, ½ cup	173			★	■	░								▒						▒	
Mashed (with milk and butter), ½ cup	98				▒	░								░						■	
POTATO CHIPS, 10	115			★		■					░									▒	
POTATO SALAD, ½ cup	125				▒									▒		▒				■	
RADISHES, 4	5													░							
SAUERKRAUT, ½ cup	20					■								■						■	
SPINACH: Cooked, ½ cup	20					▒	■				▒			■	▒			░			▒
Raw (chopped), 1 cup	15					▒	■				▒			■				▒			
SQUASH: Summer (boiled), ½ cup	15					░								░							
Winter (baked), ½ cup	65					■	■							■							■
SWEET POTATOES: Boiled, 1 medium	170				■	■	■							■				▒			
Candied, 3 oz.	175				■	▒	■														
TOMATO CATSUP, 1 tbsp.	15																			▒	
TOMATO JUICE, 1 cup	45				▒	░	■			░				■				▒		■	■
TOMATOES: Canned, ½ cup	25					░	▒							■						░	
Fresh, 1 medium	25					▒	▒							■							▒
TURNIPS, ½ cup	18					■								■							░

Bibliography

BOOKS

Adams, Catherine F., *Nutritive Value of American Foods*. U.S. Dept. of Agriculture, 1975.

Arlin, Marian, *The Science of Nutrition*. Macmillan, 1977.

Bender, Arnold E., *Food Processing and Nutrition*. Academic Press, 1978.

Briggs, George M., *Bogert's Nutrition and Physical Fitness*. W. B. Saunders, 1979.

Brody, Jane, *Jane Brody's Nutrition Book*. W. W. Norton, 1981.

Bruch, Hilde:
Eating Disorders. Basic Books, 1973.
The Golden Cage. Harvard University Press, 1978.

Deutsch, Ronald, *The New Nuts among the Berries*. Bull Publishing, 1977.

Dubos, Rene, *Man Adapting*. Yale University Press, 1965.

Goodhart, Robert S., *Modern Nutrition in Health and Disease*. Lea & Febiger, 1980.

Guthrie, Helen Andrews, *Introductory Nutrition*. C. V. Mosby, 1979.

Harris, Leslie J., *Vitamins in Theory and Practice*. Cambridge University Press, 1955.

Harris, Robert S., *Nutritional Evaluation of Food Processing*. AVI Publishing, 1975.

Herbert, Victor, *Nutrition Cultism: Facts and Fiction*. George F. Stickley, 1980.

Labuza, Theodore P., *Food and Your Well-Being*. West Publishing, 1977.

Lappé, Frances Moore, *Diet for a Small Planet*. Ballantine Books, 1975.

Leach, Penelope, *Your Baby and Child*. Knopf, 1977.

Lowenberg, Miriam E., *Food and Man*. John Wiley & Sons, 1968.

Mayer, Jean, *A Diet for Living*. Pocket Books, 1975.

McCollum, Elmer Verner, *A History of Nutrition*. Houghton Mifflin, 1957.

National Research Council, *Recommended Dietary Allowances*. National Academy of Sciences, 1980.

Nizel, Abraham E., *Nutrition in Preventive Dentistry*. W. B. Saunders, 1981.

Orr, M. L. *Amino Acid Content of Foods*. U.S. Dept. of Agriculture, 1968.

Passmore, R., *Handbook of Human Nutritional Requirements*. Food and Agriculture Organization of the United Nations, 1974.

Peckman, Gladys C., *Foundations of Food Preparation*. Macmillan, 1979.

Pennington, Jean A. T., *Food Values of Portions Commonly Used*. Harper & Row, 1980.

Posati, Linda P., *Composition of Foods*. U.S. Dept. of Agriculture, 1980.

Powers, Pauline S., *Obesity: The Regulation of Weight*. Williams & Wilkins, 1980.

Root, Waverley, and Richard de Rochemont, *Eating in America*. William Morrow, 1976.

Scarpa, Ioannis S., *Sourcebook on Food and Nutrition*. Marquis Academic Media, 1980.

Select Committee on Nutrition and Human Needs: United States Senate, *Dietary Goals for the United States*. U.S. Government Printing Office, 1977.

Spock, Dr. Benjamin, *Baby and Child Care*. Pocket Books, 1976.

Stunkard, Albert J., *Obesity*. W. B. Saunders, 1980.

Traisman, Howard S., *Management of Juvenile Diabetes Mellitus*. C. V. Mosby, 1980.

U.S. Dept. of Agriculture, *Nutritive Value of Foods*. U.S. Dept. of Agriculture, 1977.

West, Kelly M., *Epidemiology of Diabetes and its Vascular Lesions*. Elsevier North-Holland, 1978.

PERIODICALS

Adelman, Bob, "The Diet." *Esquire,* June 1980.

Bayless, Theodore M., et al., "When You Suspect Lactose Intolerance." *Patient Care,* July 15, 1980.

"Claims of Great Longevity Exaggerated." *Science News,* 106, 7, August 17, 1974.

Ember, Lois R., "Nitrosamines: Assessing the Relative Risk." *Chemical and Engineering News,* March 31, 1980.

Hardwick, J. L., "The Incidence and Distribution of Caries Throughout the Ages in Relation to the Englishman's Diet." *British Dental Journal,* 108, 1, January 5, 1960.

Hoover, Robert, "Saccharin—Bitter Aftertaste?" *The New England Journal of Medicine,* 302, 10, March 6, 1980.

Knittle, Jerome L., and Jules Hirsch, "Effect of Early Nutrition on the Development of Rat Epididymal Fat Pads: Cellularity and Metabolism." *The Journal of Clinical Investigation,* 47, 2091, September 1968.

Knittle, Jerome L., et al., "The Growth of Adipose Tissue in Children and Adolescents." *The Journal of Clinical Investigation,* 63, 239, February 1979.

May, Charles D., "Food Allergy: Perspective, Principles, Practical Management." *Nutrition Today,* November/December 1980.

Olney, John W., "Excitatory Neurotoxins as Food Additives: An Evaluation of Risk." *Neurotoxicology,* 2, 163-192, 1981.

Quensel, Carl-Erik, et al., "The Vipeholm Dental Caries Study." *Acta Odontological Scandinavica,* 2, 1954.

Van Rensburg, S. J., et al., "Circumstances Associated with the Contamination of Food by Aflatoxin in a High Primary Liver Cancer Area." *SA Medical Journal,* 49, 877, May 24, 1975.

Winick, Myron, ed., "Obesity." *Nutrition and Health,* 1, 2, 1979.

Wynder, Ernst L., "Nutritional Carcinogenesis." *Annals of New York Academy of Sciences,* 300, 360, 1977.

OTHER PUBLICATIONS

Diabetes Mellitus. Eli Lilly and Company, 1980.

Diet and Hyperactivity: Any Connection? Institute of Food Technologists, April 1976.

Dietary Salt. Institute of Food Technologists, January 1980.

Food Consumption, Prices, and Expenditures. U.S. Dept. of Agriculture, July 1968.

Foodborne Disease. Centers for Disease Control, U.S. Dept. of Health and Human Services, Annual Summary 1978, (Revised) Reissued February 1981.

Foodborne Illness. American Medical Association, December 1976.

Shelf Life of Foods. Institute of Food Technologists, August 1974.

Picture credits

Thomas S. England. 65: Cliché Musées Nationaux, Paris, courtesy Musée du Louvre. 68: J. Regunberg, courtesy Biology Department, Vassar College; inset, Jerry Calvin, courtesy Biology Department, Vassar College. 70: Courtesy Dr. Michael Stock, St. George's Hospital Medical School, London. 72: Drawing by Joan McGurren. 75: The Greenhouse. 76: Rancho La Puerta, Tecate, Baja California, Mexico. 77: Bäder- und Kurverwaltung, Baden-Baden. 82-88: © 1979 Bob Adelman. 89: © 1979 Bob Adelman—courtesy Weight Control Unit, Obesity Research Center, St. Luke's-Roosevelt Hospital Center. 90, 91: © 1979 Bob Adelman. 93: Aldo Tutino. 95: © 1974 Lennart Nilsson, from *Behold Man*, Little, Brown and Co. 99: Burt Glinn from Magnum, courtesy Bristol-Myers Co. 101: WHO photo by N. Willard; Lehtikuva Oy, Helsinki. 102, 103: Dr. S. J. van Rensburg, courtesy The National Research Institute for Nutritional Diseases, Cape Province, South Africa. 104: WHO photo by Erich Schwab. 106: Auto-Syringe, Inc. 107: Enrico Ferorelli. 108: James Cowlin from Image Enterprises. 110-117: Enrico Ferorelli. 119: Manfred Kage from Peter Arnold, Inc. 121: Enrico Ferorelli. 123: Library of Congress. 124: Courtesy H. J. Heinz Co. 125: Library of Congress. 128: Courtesy General Foods Corporation and Hillwood Museum, Washington, D.C. 132: Joe Munroe from Photo Researchers. 134-145: John Senzer. 147: Richard Jeffery. 150, 151: Kenneth Lee. 156: Centers for Disease Control, Atlanta. 159-170: Richard Jeffery.

Acknowledgments

The index for this book was prepared by Barbara L. Klein. For their help in the preparation of this volume, the editors wish to thank the following: Sidney Abraham, National Center for Health Statistics, U.S. Department of Health and Human Services, Hyattsville, Md.; Kate Alfriend, Office of Governmental and Public Affairs, U.S. Department of Agriculture (USDA), Washington, D.C.; Herman L. Amman, University of Maryland, College Park; Dr. Reubin Andres, National Institute of Aging, Baltimore; William Arthur, Hooksett, N.H.; Judith Bale, National Academy of Sciences, Washington, D.C.; Dr. Theodore M. Bayless, Johns Hopkins University Hospital, Baltimore; Sovan K. Bhattacharjee, University of Maryland, College Park; Bob Bjork, Science and Education Administration (SEA), USDA, Washington, D.C.; Dr. Per Björntörp, St. Luke's-Roosevelt Hospital Center, New York City; Dr. S. Allan Bock, Boulder, Colo.; Dr. George A. Bray, University of California at Los Angeles-Harbor Medical Center, Torrance, Calif.; George M. Briggs, University of California at Berkeley; Myrtle L. Brown, National Academy of Sciences, Washington, D.C.; Dr. Hilde Bruch, Baylor College of Medicine, Houston; Dr. John D. Brunzell, University of Washington, Seattle; Brother Henri Capdeville, Holy Trinity Monastery, St. David, Ariz.; Leon A. Carrier, The Montgomery Farm Woman's Cooperative Market Inc., Bethesda, Md.; Renée Cassaigne, Ministère de la Santé, Paris; Noreen Chen, Self-Help for the Elderly, San Francisco; Lucy Cooney, The Golden Door, Escondido, Calif.; Emil Corwin, Food and Drug Administration (FDA), Washington, D.C.; Jacques des Courtils, Ministère de la Santé, Paris; Frances J. Cronin, USDA, Washington, D.C.; Jill S. Cury, The Greenhouse, Arlington, Tex.; Dutch Food Information Bureau, Amsterdam; Dr. Donnell D. Etzwiler, Diabetes Education Center, Minneapolis; The Food and Agricultural Organization of the United Nations, Rome; André François, C.N.E.R.N.A., Paris; Jean-Luc Gianardi, Ministère de l'Agriculture, Paris; Robert Gravani, Cornell University, Ithaca, N.Y.; M.R.C. Greenwood, Vassar College, Poughkeepsie, N.Y.; Judith A. Griffin, Diabetes Education Center, Minneapolis; Janet Kolmer Grommet, Arlington, Va.; Helen Andrews Guthrie, Pennsylvania State University, University Park; Vera Haile, Self-Help for the Elderly, San Francisco; Dr. A. S. Härö, National Board of Health, Helsinki; Father Louis B. Hasenfuss, Holy Trinity Monastery, St. David, Ariz.; D. Mark Hegsted, SEA, USDA, Washington, D.C.; Frank Hepburn, SEA, USDA, Hyattsville, Md.; Dr. Jules Hirsch, The Rockefeller University, New York City; Joanne M. Holden, Beltsville Human Nutrition Center, Beltsville, Md.; Matthias Horst, Bonn; Linda Inman, Human Nutrition Center, SEA, USDA, Grand Forks, N.D.; Shichiro Ishikawa, National Cancer Center, Tokyo; Dr. Henry A. Jordan, Institute for Behavioral Education, King of Prussia, Pa.; Ruth Jordan, Baden-Baden; Dr. Charles Kaelber, National Institute on Alcohol Abuse and Alcoholism, Rockville, Md.; Endel Karmas, Kendall Park, N.J.; Richard E. Keesey, University of Wisconsin, Madison; Dr. Jerome L. Knittle, Mount Sinai School of Medicine, New York City; Paul Lachance, Princeton, N.J.; Karen Lechowich, American Dietetic Association, Chicago; Pierre Llobet, Secrétaire Général, F.I.C.U.R., Paris; David L. Margules, Temple University, Philadelphia; Jean-Yves Martin, Ministère de l'Agriculture, Paris; Howard Mattson, Institute of Food Technologists, Chicago; Dr. Charles May, Quichee, Vt.; Judith L. McBride, Beltsville Agricultural Research Center, USDA, Beltsville, Md.; Dr. Walter Mertz, Beltsville Human Nutrition Research Center, USDA, Beltsville, Md.; Corbin I. Miles, FDA, Washington, D.C.; Mary K. Moss, Beltsville Human Nutrition Center, USDA, Beltsville, Md.; Odilé Neel, Comité François d'Éducation pour la Santé, Paris; Dr. Rosemarie Neüssel, Bonn; Dr. John W. Olney, Washington University School of Medicine, St. Louis; Dr. David M. Paige, Johns Hopkins University, Baltimore; Dee Pattee, Munich; Greg Pontzious, The Heritage, San Francisco; Professor Pekka Puska, M.D., Central Laboratory of Public Health, Helsinki; Wayne D. Rasmussen, Agricultural History Branch, USDA, Washington, D.C.; Dr. Gerald Reaven, Stanford University School of Medicine, Stanford, Calif.; Dr. Arlene Redmond, St. Luke's Obesity Research Center, New York City; Dr. Judy Reid, Tucson, Ariz.; Dr. Harold Sandstead, SEA, USDA, Grand Forks, N.D.; Professor Arje Scheinin, University of Turku, Finland; Anthony Sclafani, Brooklyn College of the City University of New York; James H. Shaw, Harvard School of Dental Medicine, Boston; Dr. Jeremiah Stamler, Northwestern University, Chicago; Roger Stevens, The Heritage, San Francisco; Dr. Albert J. Stunkard, University of Pennsylvania, Philadelphia; Dr. Edward A. Sweeney, Harvard School of Dental Medicine, Boston; Deborah Szekely, Tecate, Calif.; Dr. Theodore Van Itallie, St. Luke's Obesity Research Center, New York City; Dr. S. J. Van Rensburg, National Research Institute for Nutritional Diseases, Cape Province, South Africa; Dr. A.R.P. Walker, South Africa Institute for Medical Research, Johannesburg; Nina Walter, Lancaster Beauty Farm, Baden-Baden; Dr. John H. Weisburger, American Health Foundation, Valhalla, N.Y.; Dr. Dennis Westoff, University of Maryland, College Park; Alice Whittemore, Stanford University Medical School, Stanford, Calif.; Bill Wood, Harrison, Me.; Dr. Ernst L. Wynder, American Health Foundation, New York City; Vernon R. Young, Massachusetts Institute of Technology, Cambridge; Dr. William J. Zimmermann, Iowa State University, Ames.

Index